SLEEP
WITH
THE
ANGELS

A Mother
Challenges
AIDS

SLEEP
WITH
THE
ANGELS

A Mother
Challenges
AIDS

Mary Fisher

MOYER BELL: WAKEFIELD, RHODE ISLAND & LONDON

Published by Moyer Bell

Mary Fisher's Family AIDS Network, Inc., is a nonprofit organization dedicated to increasing awareness, compassion and resources with which to fight the HIV/AIDS epidemic in America.

First Edition

**LIBRARY OF CONGRESS
CATALOGING-IN-PUBLICATION DATA**

Fisher, Mary Davis, 1948-
Sleep with the angels: A mother challenges AIDS /
Mary Davis Fisher.—1st ed.

p. cm.
1. AIDS (Disease) 2. AIDS (Disease)-Social aspects.
3. AIDS (Disease)—United States. I. Title.
RC607.A26F56   1994
362.1'969792—dc20   93-27216
ISBN: 1-55921-105-9 (cloth)   C I P
          1-55921-103-2 (paper)

Front cover photograph © 1992 *Los Angeles Times*

Printed in the United States of America
Distributed in North America by Publishers Group West, P.O. Box 8843, Emeryville CA 94662 800-788-3123 (in California 510-658-3453) and in Europe by Gazelle Book Services Ltd., Falcon House, Queen Square, Lancaster LA1 1RN England.

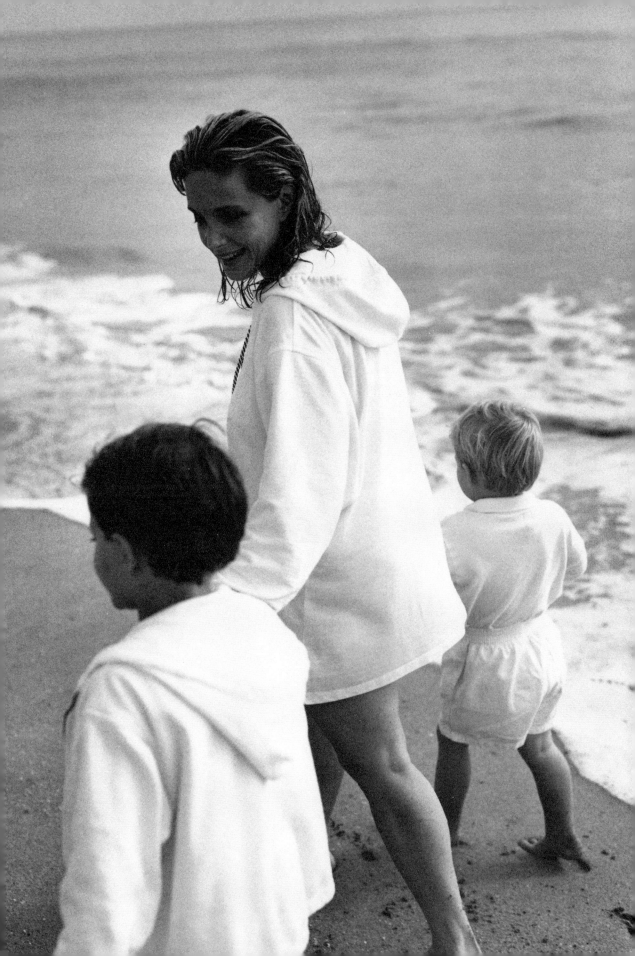

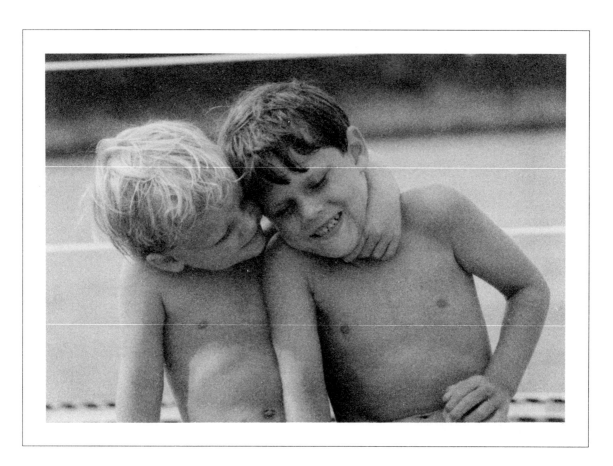

To my children, who are my inspiration and my motivation, and to your Dad, the brightest star in your sky.

CONTENTS

PHOTO CREDITS

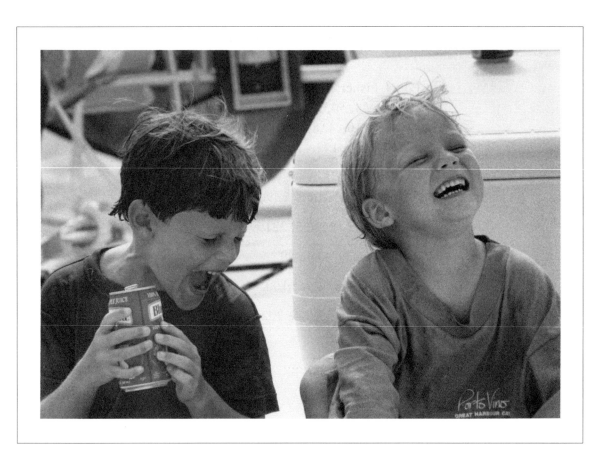

Acknowledgments

———————O———————

The photographs and speeches filling these pages sample both my public comments and my private life in recent months. They may also offer convincing evidence that my children, Max and Zachary, occupy the central place in my life.

Speeches excerpted here were not originally written to be read in a book; they were prepared to be spoken to an audience. Most photographs were meant to capture personal memories. Now both are being published—which gives me the opportunity to name some of those who've helped shape what has become a publication.

Thousands of usually unpaid and unheralded volunteers, many active in local AIDS organizations, conceived, planned and sponsored events which led to speeches that now appear here. I cannot name them all, but if they had never asked me to speak—and encouraged me to speak candidly—most of what's written in the following pages would never have been composed.

From the first time my story was told publicly, my ability to pursue a mission of awareness and compassion has depended on a fragile and seldom-acknowledged partnership with media: national, regional, and local. Without journalists and reporters to cover and retell the story with sensitivity and dignity, the story would have reached thousands instead of millions. Producers and editors who created space in broadcasts and on editorial pages, and then filled that space with a sometimes unpopular message, set a pattern which was more important than my few moments in their limelights. From an hour of joyful hysteria in a television studio in Salt Lake City to a moment of gripping grief in an art gallery in Florida; from stagehands at ABC who asked me to sign their wall to network anchors who encouraged me to "say it again"—the hardworking and sometimes maligned professionals known collectively as "the media," who've covered these speeches from city to city, have earned my appreciation and this brief acknowledgment.

Behind the scenes, friends and heroes have offered everything from loving criticism to extraordinary support. The name of Betty Ford is the first that comes to mind. No matter what the hour of the day or the issue at hand, she's been ready to offer wise counsel and steady encouragement. And then come other names: Jeanne Ashe, who has taught all of us about courage and purpose; Sally Fisher, who saw my naivete as a challenge and met it with strength and humor; Bob Larson, whose convictions and compassion are deeper than anyone may ever know; Dr. Henry Murray, whose concern for his patients is wrapped in love as well as science; and Dr. June Osborn who, when first she heard my story, swept into my life with hope and friendship.

As the pages of this book show, I hate the AIDS virus although I'm grateful for the meaning of my life. Finding and maintaining the balance between this hatred and this gratitude can sometimes by tricky. When perspective begins to slip, I've often turned to the members of my "AIDS family," exceptional people who share a passionate distaste for the virus that ravages our lives and the lives of others we love. Michael Iskowitz sends funny cartoons and insightful suggestions; Larry Kramer proves that integrity is something we have, not something others can give (or take from) us; Dr. David Rogers offers a wisdom and grace that redeem our worst days; Jeffrey Schmalz shows how to maintain vulnerability without self-pity—and the list goes on.

The discovery that we are HIV-positive tends to divide our lives into "before" and "after." Some friends and family members bridged these two eras of my life with special grace: Joy Anderson and Joy Prouty, Henry Baskin and Byron Nease, Judy Sherman and Stu White, Kathie Durham and Anne Keating, Geoff Mason and Brian Weiss, and extraordinary members of my family— especially my parents, whose concern has been constant; my brother, Phillip, who shows his love in part by helping lead the Family AIDS Network and by helping me through the hardest hours; my sister-in-law, Tina Campbell, whose love for a dying brother never excluded Max or Zack or me; and my cousin Dr. Michael Saag whose pioneer research in Alabama may be the fountain from which the world's first effective AIDS treatment flows.

Patty Presock lives by the maxim, "Do the right thing," and has encouraged me and others to follow that same advice. Having given such wise guidance, she then gave us another gift, her daugher, Tracy, now working fulltime for the Family AIDS Network. Tracy, first in Florida and more recently in Washington, D.C., and the staff of The Greystone Group in Grand Rapids, Michigan, provide day-to-day staffing distinguished by flexibility, hard work and excellence. Fielding and managing everything from crisis telephone calls to faltering airline schedules, these colleagues have proven that a small group of people can, when thoroughly committed to the mission, move a whole range of mountains.

Jennifer Moyer and Britt Bell lent more than the name of their publishing company to this effort; they poured themselves into the project. As it headed for press, they put my name and picture on the cover. But I think of it as belonging to them, and to all those named above. Most of all, I think of this book as belonging to my children. If it were not for them, I could not have the passion that has produced this book.

Without the contributions of two special colleagues, this book might have had its passion but not its potency. David Hume Kennerly—who persuaded me first to buy a real camera and then to risk, as an artist, publishing my work here—has won the Pulitzer with his photojournalism, my heart with his readiness to embrace each new day, and my gratitude for his help in shaping this book. And A. James Heynen, who came into my life like a gift of God, able to translate my soul (even when it is mute) into words that have stirred the souls of others. . .for him, I have no words.

To all of these—and to all those I should have thanked but could not—my gratitude. And, beyond my gratitude, my love.

SLEEP
WITH
THE
ANGELS

A Mother
Challenges
AIDS

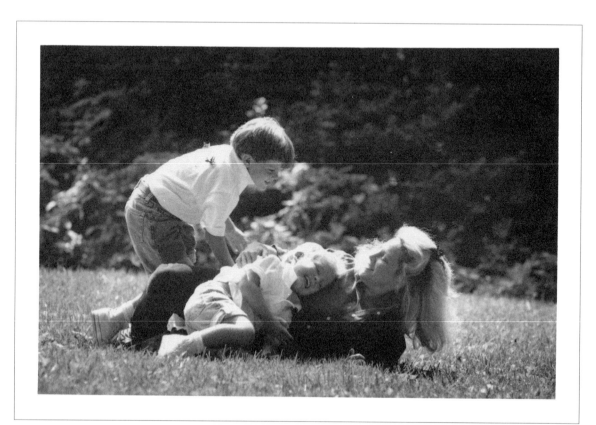

A Letter to My Children

---o---

Mothers' Voices Luncheon
New York City
May 4, 1992

I learned that I was HIV-positive in July 1991. After months of agonizing questions and hard conversations, in February, 1992, I told my story in public. A few weeks later, Georgette Mosbacher called to ask if I would accept a tribute from the American Foundation for AIDS Research (AmFAR), their "Award of Courage." I was honored. Then, after I'd accepted her invitation, I heard her add: "Mathilde [Krim, AmFAR President] would like you to give a few remarks." Now I was honored and terrified. I had never given a public speech in my adult life. I'd been a television producer, a White House advanceman, an artist—but never a public speaker.

While worrying about the AmFAR speech I met a remarkable man, Jim ("A. James") Heynen. As president of a consult-

19

ing firm, The Greystone Group, he'd advised corporate execu- tives and public figures for years. But in the quiet of my home he gave me the simplest counsel: "Don't worry about a speech, just tell the truth in public. If you can be vulnerable, you will be powerful." Within a week, we'd become partners in the mis- sion. I'd tell him the truth and he'd draft words to communicate that truth to others. Beginning with "A Letter to My Children," every speech I've given—every paragraph in this book— resulted from our collaboration. Jim listens to my soul and gives it a public voice.

Although I am by profession an artist, my day-to-day struggle with AIDS is most defined by my role as a mother who never imagined she could be HIV-positive. When I went public, I had decided (as I told the AmFAR audience) "that I should not run and hide. I should stand up and fight, occasionally with tears but mostly with love." And so, when I was asked to speak "from mother to mother" at a luncheon in New York City, it seemed natural that I should read something expressing that love: A letter to my children.

Dear Max and Zack,

You're sleeping now at last . . . .

Some days I think this nighttime peace will never come. I love my days with you. Your reliable smile was the only thing that lit up this frantic house today, Max. And, Zachary, I sometimes think that if I had half your energy and persistence, I'd accomplish miracles in minutes. But loving my days with you as I do, I have a motherly confession to make—I love the hour you fall asleep as well.

It's a delicious time. A quiet time. For those few minutes, I will not hear the word I love most: "Mom!" I just visited your rooms to pull the covers over each of you and thought how blessed I am, not only to have you, but to have you asleep.

Often at this time of night I write in your journals, the ones I've been keeping for each of you since you were born. You see, it wasn't enough to just record your first haircuts, steps and words. I wanted you to know how I felt about those monumental moments as well as what I fear most.

You're children and I'm an adult but by the time you read this letter, you'll be adults too—and I'll no longer be the young mother I am now. So you could know, as an adult, who your Mom is—I've kept your journals.

I've not said much in your journals about "being positive," about the swirl of publicity and confusion and the weariness that has accompanied our last year. Usually by this time of night I've had all of that I can stand. I want to return to being a Mom or an artist or a friend. I'm tired of being "The AIDS Person." I want to be me for a little while.

Tomorrow I must leave you again for another trip to visit with important people about important things. It's all very, very important. And I wish I were with you—because you, Max and Zack, are the most important to me.

People will ask me questions about AIDS. And I will answer the questions again, as I've answered them a hundred times before. But what I would really like to say is based on something small and simple . . . us.

I'm eager to go out in the world with the message that "If Mary Fisher can get AIDS, so can you." I'll happily donate time to the causes that could enable me to attend your high school graduation.

But I'm also eager to stay home. Because I'm keenly aware, in ways I never imagined, of the consequences this illness has had, is having, and will have on our family. We have, all of us, now discovered what hundreds of thousands of American families discovered before us:

AIDS does more than kill bodies. It destroys families.

The single hardest day of my life was not the day I heard my test results. Stunning as that was—standing at LaGuardia airport with you two playing nearby, getting the news from an apologetic stranger—more difficult by far was the day I needed to tell your grandfather the truth about AIDS in his family. I did not fear my dying from the disease at that moment. I feared how he might live with the truth. It took me weeks to come to grips with the reality. I kept saying to myself, "This isn't possible. This can't be real." It took me months to move from shock to anger to hurt to grief to surrender and acceptance—and only recently, to effective action.

Once I had accepted the truth, I expected everyone else would accept it too. I was totally unprepared for the reality that everyone who loved me would go through every stage I'd gone through.

If they were shocked and angry, I assumed they were angry with me, because I had this dread disease. I hadn't even known I was at risk. But when they faced prejudice and stigma because of my condition, I felt guilty, as if I had done something wrong.

What I know today, Max and Zack, is more than I knew a year ago. Your grandparents, your uncles and aunts and our extended family of relatives and friends, they have rallied around us with affection and commitment as quickly as they were able. Much as I needed to endure the process, they, too, wrestled with their own griefs, confronted their own feelings of anger and shame, and moved again to tighten the bands of unconditional love that hold us together as a family.

If I have not told you so before, let me say it to you plainly now. Max and Zack, I not only love you wildly, I need you. I need my family. I need you and everyone else more now than I ever have before. And sometimes when I look too far in the future, I realize how much I will need you then.

But when fear becomes a poison, threatening to rob us of the joy we had rolling on the floor, tickling each other and laughing today, the antidote is us, our family. So long as we have family— you and I—all of us will go on.

Tonight when I tucked each of you into bed, I said to you what you've heard me say every night of your lives. Since the moment you came from my body, Max, and the hour you were placed in my arms, Zachary, I have known that I would, one day, need to give you up.

And so, each night, I rehearse for the day when I must give you over. That is why as I reach for the day's last kiss and hug, you always hear me say the same four words,

"Sleep with the angels . . . ."

Love,
Mom

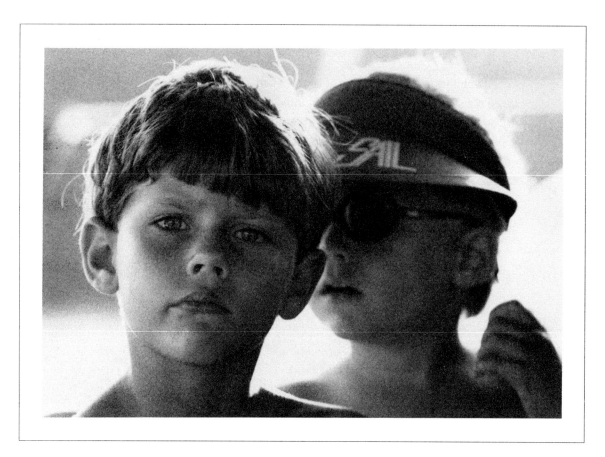

The Shroud of Silence

---O---

Republican Platform Committee
Salt Lake City
May 26, 1992

When I went public, I wanted to make a difference. But I genuinely had no idea how that would happen. The Detroit Free Press, *my hometown newspaper, published the first account of my story. Then came the AmFAR award and some more media. Before long, my telephone was ringing.*

My father had been strong and supportive from the day I told him I was HIV-positive. That his daughter was on the road to AIDS was frustrating enough; that it seemed impossible for him to do anything about it was worse. Because 1992 was a presidential election year, and because he was active in the campaign, I think he was pleased when I told him I was scheduled to testify at platform hearings in Utah.

I went alone to Salt Lake City where, in the heart of that beautiful city, I felt like an alien. I knew no one and hardly knew myself. The platform hearings were loaded with tightly-timed presentations from people armed with charts and graphs and plenty of ammunition to attack taxes and spending. Not only was I the only one wearing a red (AIDS Awareness) ribbon; I imagined I was the only one there who knew what it represented. I had no charts, no graphs, and no second-string if I should falter: All I had was my father's name and my own story.

Late in the afternoon, Senator Donald Nickles (R-Oklahoma) introduced my fellow-panelists and me. I watched the C-SPAN cameraman while others spoke. Then it was my turn to speak—the first but not the last time I felt like "the only HIV-positive Republican."

I am grateful to be here today and also to represent the tradition of my father, Max Fisher, Honorary Chairman of the Bush/Quayle '92 National Finance Committee. It is his hope and mine that the Republican Party will adopt a position of leadership in the face of America's most threatening epidemic.

I was raised in a home which prepared me for a career in the arts, in television production and especially in service to my community and my country. What none of us were prepared for was the news last July that I had tested HIV-positive. Max Fisher's daughter, a married woman, my children's mother—who never knew she was at risk—I am on the road to AIDS. That is one reason I am speaking to you today.

Another reason is that I am, like my father, a lifelong Republican. I've served from the privacy of my home to the White House, where I was the first woman "Advanceman" for another Republican President, Gerald Ford. This party has my loyalty.

You know the historic statistics concerning AIDS: It has infected over a million Americans and killed more of us than all the wars in this century. But I want to speak to you of the future which is even more alarming. In the past, we thought of this as "their" disease. . . whoever "they" were. We cannot do that now, and we will never be able to do that again. This is not "their disease," it is "ours." It is spreading fastest among adolescents, women and children. In that regard, I am typical. I am not a special-interest group and this is not a special-interest disease. The difference between AIDS and other leading killers is that AIDS is a communicable plague. You cannot catch heart disease; cancer is not contagious. But AIDS cuts across all traditional boundaries: race and age, community and class, even all other diseases.

At Notre Dame's commencement a few days ago, President Bush observed that political "parties, like people, have tendencies." In the arena of AIDS, we Republicans have shown two tendencies.

First, in point of fact, we have supported bipartisan programs for research and education, for prevention and for care. Even so, we recognize in the face of this wildfire epidemic that much more is urgently needed.

Second, we have shown a tendency to be quiet. Perhaps we are uncertain what to say, or how to say it. For whatever reason, we have taken refuge in silence. To those fifteen million Americans whose homes and lives are already gripped by AIDS, ours is a thundering silence.

Today I am asking you to help us, as Republicans and as Americans, to lift our shroud of silence and speak with the voice of compassion.

The epidemic is too vast to give it a mere sliver in the platform. The cry for leadership cannot be answered by a quick whisper. If we launch this campaign beneath our shroud of silence, no one will believe we are a party of either courage or compassion. And I have been raised to believe we are both.

Let me be clear: I would happily forfeit my role in this drama. I love my children and would like to see them grown. I never imagined I would be here in such a position. But I have learned the lesson you must learn. It doesn't matter that I'm not gay; it doesn't matter that I'm not hemophiliac; it doesn't matter that I'm not an IV-drug user. None of this matters because I am not the past of this disease. I am its future. If you believe, as I did, that you and your children are not at risk, then take home this lesson from me: You are.

Throughout this past year, President and Mrs. Bush have been an affectionate source of support for me and my family. We are grateful for their love. But you must let their voice of private compassion become our voice of public leadership. We do the President no favor by leaving in place the Republican shroud of silence, encouraging millions in AIDS-affected families to believe that they must turn elsewhere to hear a voice of genuine compassion.

Since publicly disclosing my HIV status in February, 1992, I've answered hard and intimate questions before television cameras and in the press. But the hardest questions have come not from seasoned journalists but from my family. My sons, who are too young to understand about living and dying, have found me in quiet and vulnerable moments. Max asked why I cry; Zachary asked if he could bring me his "night-night." My father, who has spent decades helping the nations, wants to know how to heal his daughter; he can't. My brother and mother, sisters and friends have asked what they can do. In large measure, the answer is, there's little they can do.

But you can. You can lift our party's suffocating shroud of silence by putting a strong statement in our platform which unambiguously recognizes AIDS as a family disease. As the party committed to the healing of the American family, let us demonstrate:

First, that we have the will to provide national leadership in the face of this mounting tragedy;

Second, that we have the commitment to support accurate and candid education which will slow the growth of the escalating epidemic;

Third, that we have the insight to mount an effective campaign for research;

Fourth, that we have the concern to care for individuals and families broken by this illness; and,

Finally, that because we love justice we will defend the sick and dying against stigma and discrimination.

Such a statement will lift our shroud of silence, speak boldly in a voice of compassion, and do justice to the tradition which brought us all here today. I wish you wisdom and courage.

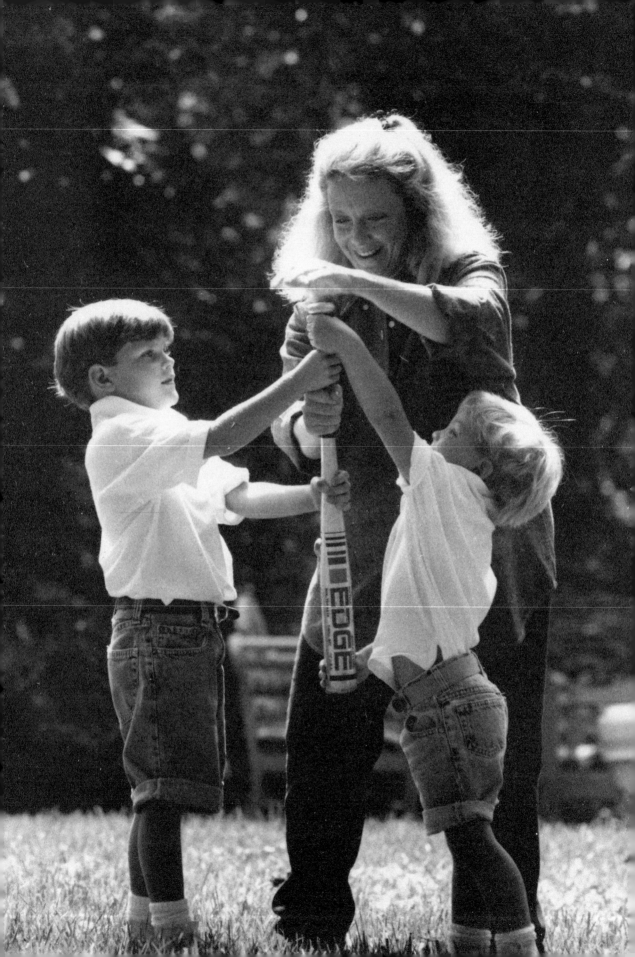

A Mother's Call to Partnership

---O---

VIII International Conference on
AIDS/HIV STD World Congress
Amsterdam, The Netherlands
July 23, 1992

*A year after the telephone call which told me I was HIV-
positive, I received a call inviting me to speak in The Netherlands at the VIII International Conference on AIDS/HIV STD
World Congress. My mother, who had helped me deal with the
first of these calls, agreed to accompany me in response to the
second. We took on Amsterdam together.*

*Mother has traveled the world but attended very few
conferences. As we headed for Amsterdam, she clearly had
expectations which were bound to turn into disappointments.
She could not imagine that something as prestigious as an
International Conference—a "World Congress," it said in the
brochures!—could provide anything less than a cure. Mother*

was going to Amsterdam to hear an announcement that wasn't going to be made. Quite the contrary: She wound up spending intense days, and equally intense nights, with people struggling to remain hopeful in the face of news that justified less and less hope. It may have been here, a year after she first heard the news, that mother came to grips with the meaning of my infection.

For me, Amsterdam was the place in which I learned how large my family—my "AIDS Family"—really was. And it was with that discovery that I began my remarks.

I think of myself as a veteran in most settings which involve politics or the media, both of which are amply present at this Conference. But this week, more than ever, I've felt keenly my status as a rookie. I am a newcomer. I'm new both to the anger and frustration and to the support and affection which flow through this Conference. I've spent the past year dealing with quiet grief, not global policy. I'm more mother than crusader; I cling to my children in the night.

You've asked about my experience. Let me begin here, in Amsterdam, where I've discovered in the past few days that all differences are flattened by HIV. We share residence in a global village and membership in a global family. Although this family is divided by nation and race, gender and economy, once we are HIV-positive, the divisions fade. Suddenly I am one with the child who walks the dusty roads of Nigeria, the grandmother who tends her infected family in Manila, the gay stockbroker in San Francisco and every HIV-infected mother who longs to see her children grow to adulthood. We have in common, all of us, this unwelcome disease. I am enriched by a new solidarity with brothers and sisters of many colors and places.

When the virus found me, it found an American, a mother of two children, an artist, a woman with experience in the media and the government. It found a person whose life song has been an anthem of activity: I am a do-er. I take refuge in action and cannot abide inactivity. It's a family tradition. It hurt my 84-year-old father to learn that I am HIV-positive. But what hurts him most is his inability to do anything about it, to fix it.

Some months ago I joined the public call for AIDS awareness. But awareness without action is worse than no awareness at all. To know an evil and not challenge it is worse than innocent ignorance. And this is the message we all must bear: That the world cannot love us *and* ignore us.

I have long believed that life has purpose, and my HIV-positive status has not changed this conviction. In all things, I believe, there is meaning. I'd not have chosen to be HIV-positive, but I believe I was chosen for a reason—and I believe that good can come of this evil.

Let me be clear: With HIV have come unimaginable fears and vicious pain. But also with HIV has come new and fuller meaning in my life. It has created an urgency and shaped a new message. The virus is brutal, but my life—my experience with it—is a gift. Therefore, I have learned to say to those in positions of power: "Do not pity me; listen to me. I am not a victim; I am a messenger. And the message I bring is that the world must respond to this epidemic not because I may die of it, but because millions of us are living with it."

I have long believed that each of us must do most what we do best. If you have the gift of an inquiring mind, use it; if you are given creativity, pursue it. Pick the role that fits you best, because none of us can play all the roles.

We will not always succeed, of course, and we will not always get our way. The scientists who labor for my life have not made the discovery for which they search. Elected officials who want to be responsive lack the political or financial resources with which to respond. The speech I want to give falls flat; the statistics become elusive and my audience grows restless. I understand frustration; I have enough of it myself.

But frustration when confronting a worldwide disaster is to be expected. And if it is true that we are one global family, sharing one global village, then we must move beyond our own frustrations to effective action. If I had a single plea which I would make to my brothers and sisters worldwide, it is this: Let us not be divided by our frustrations. Let us, instead, recommit ourselves to stronger, broader, and more effective partnerships.

Wiser minds than mine can speak to the intricacies of international partnerships. The only insight I have is this: Without partnerships, we will fail. With them, we can counter the epidemic's attack on every front. Those with technical knowledge must apply it; those with a moving message must deliver it; those with wealth must dedicate it; those with knowledge must teach it; those with hope must share it. We must covet cooperation and shun competition.

Perhaps my being a newcomer, or being a mother, makes me think of partnerships in personal terms. Whatever the cause, I did not come to Amsterdam merely to give a speech. I have two young sons. Their names are Max and Zachary. Unless someone produces a miracle, my children are destined to become orphans. So I've come to Amsterdam to meet those who live with me in the HIV-community.

I cannot speak every language; but if those with other tongues would give me their message, and take mine, together we can address the world. I cannot even assure my children that I will be their parent for long; but if my brothers and sisters would be my partners, I can assure my sons that the global village will wrap two more children in love.

I have come searching for those who would understand my pain and be willing to share it. I need courageous models, so I will not be discouraged while calling for change that is slow in coming. I need someone to hold me when I can no longer hold myself, to tell me the fight matters when I have no fight left within me. I need someone to say they understand, they care, they will not forget.

I have sometimes feared rejection because I am not gay, because I am not an IV-drug user, because I am not poor—or even because I am an American. But I have discovered great security in the unity which binds us.

I've told others in recent months that we must measure the value of our lives not by life's length, but by its depth. You've deepened my life in the past five days by giving me the texture of many cultures, the color of many races, the harmony of many voices, and hope.

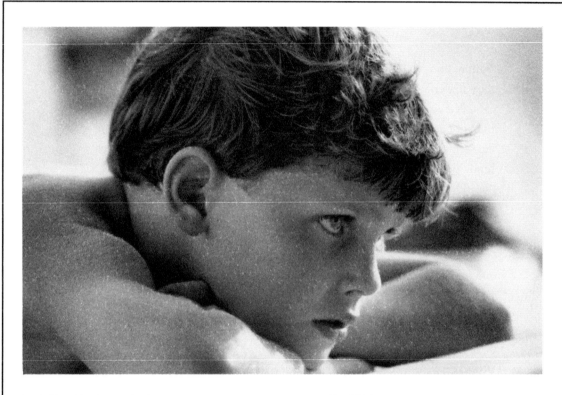

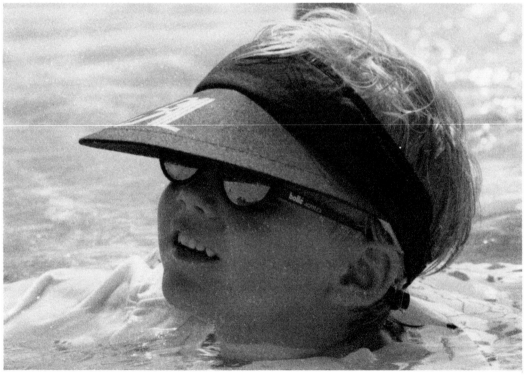

A Whisper of AIDS

———————o———————

Republican National Convention
Houston
August 19, 1992

Shortly after the Republican platform hearings in Salt Lake City, we heard rumors that I might be invited to address the August Convention. When, in July, Elizabeth Glaser and Bob Hattoy spoke about AIDS during prime broadcast time from the Democratic National Convention in New York City, the media wanted to know if the Republican leadership would even touch the issue in August. Eventually, I was invited to speak.

The weeks leading to Houston were uncomfortable. Friends in the AIDS community were (as they later confided) worried that I would say too little; friends in the Republican leadership were concerned that I would say too much. As the time grew shorter, the media grew busier. I was everywhere from The New York Times *to* USA Today *to* PEOPLE *magazine.*

The astrodome was being picketed when we arrived in Houston. ACT UP members and others were challenging the Republican record on AIDS. As the President's motorcade drove by the day before I was scheduled to speak, his car was pelted with loaded condoms. Then a protestor disrupted a news conference. The Republicans were growing edgy about AIDS.

I'd been warned to ignore the noise in the auditorium while I spoke. "They'll just walk around and talk, but don't pay any attention." So, when I started to speak, I focused on Betty Ford and the President who were seated with my family 100 feet from the podium. I watched a young man take off his shirt to reveal a T-shirt which read, "No one here knows I'm HIV-positive." Five minutes into the speech, I couldn't hear any noise: The auditorium was eerily quiet. I didn't know what was wrong, but I just kept talking. When I ended, and they came back to life in applause, I realized something good had happened: They'd listened.

Less than three months ago, at platform hearings in Salt Lake City, I asked the Republican Party to lift the shroud of silence which has been draped over the issue of HIV/AIDS. I have come tonight to bring our silence to an end.

I bear a message of challenge, not self-congratulation. I want your attention, not your applause. I would never have asked to be HIV-positive. But I believe that in all things there is a good purpose, and so I stand before you, and before the nation, gladly.

The reality of AIDS is brutally clear. Two hundred thousand Americans are dead or dying; a million more are infected. Worldwide, forty million, or sixty million, or a hundred million infections will be counted in the coming few years. But despite science and research, White House meetings and congressional hearings; despite good intentions and bold initiatives, campaign slogans and hopeful promises—despite it all, it's the epidemic which is winning tonight.

In the context of an election year, I ask you—here, in this great hall, or listening in the quiet of your home—to recognize that the AIDS virus is not a political creature. It does not care whether you are Democrat or Republican. It does not ask whether you are black or white, male or female, gay or straight, young or old.

Tonight, I represent an AIDS community whose members have been reluctantly drafted from every segment of American society. Though I am white, and a mother, I am one with a black infant struggling with tubes in a Philadelphia hospital. Though I am female, and contracted this disease in marriage, and enjoy the warm support of my family, I am one with the lonely gay man sheltering a flickering candle from the cold wind of his family's rejection.

This is not a distant threat; it is a present danger. The rate of infection is increasing fastest among women and children. Largely unknown a decade ago, AIDS is the third leading killer of young-adult Americans today—but it won't be third for long. Because, unlike other diseases, this one travels. Adolescents don't give each other cancer or heart disease because they believe they are in love. But HIV is different. And we have helped it along—we have killed each other—with our ignorance, our prejudice, and our silence.

We may take refuge in our stereotypes, but we cannot hide there long. Because HIV asks only one thing of those it attacks: Are you human? And this is the right question: Are you human? Because people with HIV have not entered some alien state of being. They are human. They have not earned cruelty and they do not deserve meanness. They don't benefit from being isolated or treated as outcasts. Each of them is exactly what God made: a person. Not evil, deserving of our judgment; not victims, longing for our pity. People. Ready for support and worthy of compassion.

My call to you, my Party, is to take a public stand no less compassionate than that of the President and Mrs. Bush. They have embraced me and my family in memorable ways. In the place of judgment, they have shown affection. In difficult moments, they have raised our spirits. In the darkest hours, I have seen them reaching not only to me, but also to my parents, armed with that stunning grief and special grace that comes only to parents who have themselves leaned too long over the bedside of a dying child.

With the President's leadership, much good has been done; much of the good has gone unheralded; as the President has insisted, "Much remains to be done."

But we do the President's cause no good if we praise the American family but ignore a virus that destroys it. We must be consistent if we are to be believed. We cannot love justice and ignore prejudice, love our children and fear to teach them. Whatever our role, as parent or policy maker, we must act as eloquently as we speak—else we have no integrity.

My call to the nation is a plea for awareness. If you believe you are safe, you are in danger. Because I was not hemophiliac, I was not at risk. Because I was not gay, I was not at risk. Because I did not inject drugs, I was not at risk.

My father has devoted much of his lifetime to guarding against another holocaust. He is part of the generation who heard Pastor Niemoeller come out of the Nazi death camps to say, "They came after the Jews and I was not a Jew, so I did not protest. They came after the Trade Unionists, and I was not a Trade Unionist, so I did not protest. They came after the Roman Catholics, and I was not a

Roman Catholic, so I did not protest. Then they came after me, and there was no one left to protest."

The lesson history teaches is this: If you believe you are safe, you are at risk. If you do not see this killer stalking your children, look again. There is no family or community, no race or religion, no place left in America that is safe. Until we genuinely embrace this message, we are a nation at risk.

Tonight, HIV marches resolutely toward AIDS in more than a million American homes, littering its pathway with the bodies of the young. Young men. Young women. Young parents. Young children. One of the families is mine. If it is true that HIV inevitably turns to AIDS, then my children will inevitably turn to orphans.

My family has been a rock of support. My 84-year-old father, who has pursued the healing of the nations, will not accept the premise that he cannot heal his daughter. My mother has refused to be broken; she still calls at midnight to tell wonderful jokes that make me laugh. Sisters and friends, and my brother Phillip (whose birthday is today)—all have helped carry me over the hardest places. I am blessed, richly and deeply blessed, to have such a family.

But not all of you have been so blessed. You are HIV-positive but dare not say it. You have lost loved ones, but you dared not whisper the word AIDS. You weep silently; you grieve alone.

I have a message for you: It is not you who should feel shame; it is we. We who tolerate ignorance and practice prejudice, we who have taught you to fear. We must lift our shroud of silence, making it safe for you to reach out for compassion. It is our task to seek safety for our children, not in quiet denial but in effective action.

Some day our children will be grown. My son Max, now four, will take the measure of his mother; my son Zachary, now two, will sort through his memories. I may not be here to hear their judgments, but I know already what I hope they are.

I want my children to know that their mother was not a victim. She was a messenger. I do not want them to think, as I once did, that courage is the absence of fear; I want them to know that courage is the strength to act wisely when most we are afraid. I want them to have the courage to step forward when called by their nation, or their Party, and give leadership—no matter what the personal cost. I ask no more of you than I ask of myself, or of my children.

To the millions of you who are grieving, who are frightened, who have suffered the ravages of AIDS firsthand: Have courage and you will find comfort.

To the millions who are strong, I issue this plea: Set aside prejudice and politics to make room for compassion and sound policy.

To my children, I make this pledge: I will not give in, Zachary, because I draw my courage from you. Your silly giggle gives me hope. Your gentle prayers give me strength. And you, my child, give me reason to say to America, "You are at risk." And I will not rest, Max, until I have done all I can to make your world safe. I will seek a place where intimacy is not the prelude to suffering.

I will not hurry to leave you, my children. But when I go, I pray that you will not suffer shame on my account.

To all within sound of my voice, I appeal: Learn with me the lessons of history and of grace, so my children will not be afraid to say the word AIDS when I am gone. Then their children, and yours, may not need to whisper it at all.

God bless the children, and bless us all.

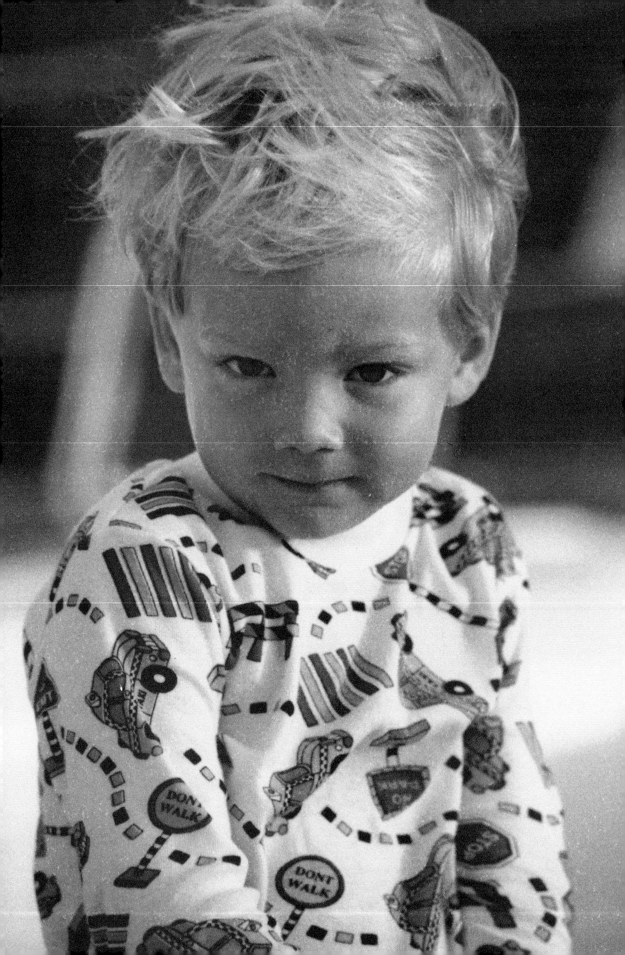

Homecoming

———————O———————

AIDS Consortium of Southeastern Michigan Dinner
Detroit
September 15, 1992

I had made no public appearances in Detroit since February when I'd told my story through the local media. So when I was invited to give a keynote to a group of Detroit AIDS careproviders, it gave me an opportunity to have my first public homecoming since the news had broken. I had some butterflies. . . .

By now, I knew what themes I wanted to stress in my speeches: compassion, dignity, courage, awareness of risk, the need for unity within the AIDS community, the promise of hope. I wanted others to realize that this disease is content to infect any human being, and that those it chooses are not somehow less human because of their infection. And I was

45

willing to be used as an example—else, why would I have gone public?

I'd discussed these themes with strangers in other places before. But I'd never given such a speech with my family and closest friends in the audience. And on this occasion, even friends from Florida (Brian Weiss and Joy Prouty, who helped me create the Family AIDS Network and were in town for the inaugural board meeting) would be in my hometown audience. For me, it was a very emotional evening—genuinely, a home-coming.

I'm grateful to be here this evening because I still think of myself as a Detroiter. This isn't a place I visit; I come home to Detroit.

Thomas Wolfe said that we can never go home again. In the sense that families and communities change, that's true. I can never return to the same group of adolescent classmates or the same production crew at WXYZ. I can't go home again—and neither can you. We are, like it or not, in a brave new world where none of us has been before.

In some respects, the tiny virus I carry is typical of this world. Unknown and unnamed barely a decade ago, today it is equally at home in the crack house and in the country club. It took ten years for AIDS to claim its first 100,000 American lives. So rapidly is the epidemic spreading that the second hundred thousand have died in a two-year span. From nursery schools to nursing homes, from bedrooms to board rooms, AIDS has changed the public agenda and private patterns which define community.

Mainly what this tiny virus does to communities is destroy them, including the most intimate community we know: our fami-lies. Nothing wreaks havoc in a family more quickly than this grim little reaper. It lays a shroud of anxiety over the future, wearing down resistance to poverty, abuse and depression until, having infected the body, AIDS destroys the family.

So, coming home to Detroit, I've discovered it isn't only the community which has changed. So have I. When I came through the kitchen door last week, I was not the person who left.

Last February was the bigger homecoming. I came home to tell you all that I was HIV-positive. What I didn't say then, and have never before now said publicly, is that I chose to go public in my hometown not because I thought it would be easiest, but because I thought it would be hardest. It seemed to me that if I could stand in public and say it here, I could stand anywhere. If my parents and brother and sisters would endure the message here, they could endure it anywhere. I thought that if rejection or condemnation were going to come, I'd prefer it at the beginning and at home. And so I went public here, holding my breath with a sense of dread.

Our experience as a family has been overwhelmingly positive. The volume of letters and calls, the promises of prayer and support, the hugs from strangers and calls from old classmates—I'd never imagined that my life would be so rich, or that I would be so surrounded by affection. Detroit has been more than a distant hometown for me since February; it has been a present source of spiritual and emotional strength.

Like everyone who is HIV-positive, I detest the condition itself. But it has its own rewards. One reward is that, by testing positive, you are inducted into a new community, the HIV/AIDS family. It's a family joined by a common fate. No matter our race or nation, gender or status, we are one: suffering the same grief, offering the same players, seeking the same answers.

There is a unity within the HIV family which defies all other divisions. But this unity is fragile. That's why the AIDS Consortium and other coalitions have taken on new importance. Because, if the HIV/AIDS community is to overcome not only illness but everything that comes with it—poverty, depression, bigotry, fear, and ignorance, to name a few—we must remain united.

There are old differences that could divide us. We are black and white, Asian and Hispanic, gay and straight. We are not all liberal or conservative, Republican or Democrat, urban or suburban. These are the things that mark us as different from one another. But they need not divide us. On the contrary: They contribute to a diverse unity which makes us stronger.

We must pay attention to what makes us unique and respect our differences. But those of us within the HIV/AIDS community have a sacred duty to preserve unity. We are not yet a community of power. As our legislative record demonstrates, we have lacked almost everything necessary to make change. Our strength is found only in this: We are one together. There is nothing worth the sacrifice of this unity. Nothing. No political gain. No legislative action. No financial or psychological edge. Nothing.

Some years ago I left my hometown alone; tonight, I've come home in the company of a million-and-a-half brothers and sisters. Not all have been graced with caring families and public support. Many so dread discovery that they live a life of terror-filled nights. They dare not whisper the word AIDS, lest in breaking their silence they lose their jobs, and in losing employment they forfeit insurance. They dare not ask for their family's embrace, lest their request become the grounds for their dismissal. They hear messages of hatred and bigotry, telling them they deserve to suffer because they have no value. What's worse, they believe such lies.

If to those within the community I appeal for unity, to those outside I appeal for acceptance. If we went home to our neighborhoods tonight, eager to open doors and hearts now closed to suffering, it would be a very good thing indeed.

My family has been showered with affection and support from all of you within this remarkable community. Therefore, we know the potential of Detroit to embrace those who fear rejection. But there are thousands here who have not yet had my experience. They are struggling to find room in this family, this home, this community: The AIDS infant who was rejected before she drew her first breath or felt her first hug; the healthy children becoming orphans because parents are HIV-positive—who will be family to them? The drug-addicted mother who cared only for escape, and now will pay with her life; the gay young man who barely knew who he was, and now knows only a wasting existence; the teenager who had so little self-esteem he took life-threatening risks, and lost—tell me: Who will be family to them?

I have come home bringing with me these brothers and sisters. If you would let me in, I am bringing company. If you would accept me, accept them. Because I, who gave one ten-minute speech to the nation, am no more worthy than a sister who cries out alone for help in a darkened alleyway. I, who became infected in marriage, am no more innocent or guilty than any other person who never wanted this disease.

So it isn't entirely true, what Thomas Wolfe wrote. I can come home. But I cannot come home alone. Now, I come in the company of those who ask that you raise high the roofbeams in this home to make room for them—to make room for all of us. It will be a home warmed by compassion, made strong with justice. It will be a place were black and white, young and the old, weak and strong—where you and I and all of us will one day say, "It is good to be home."

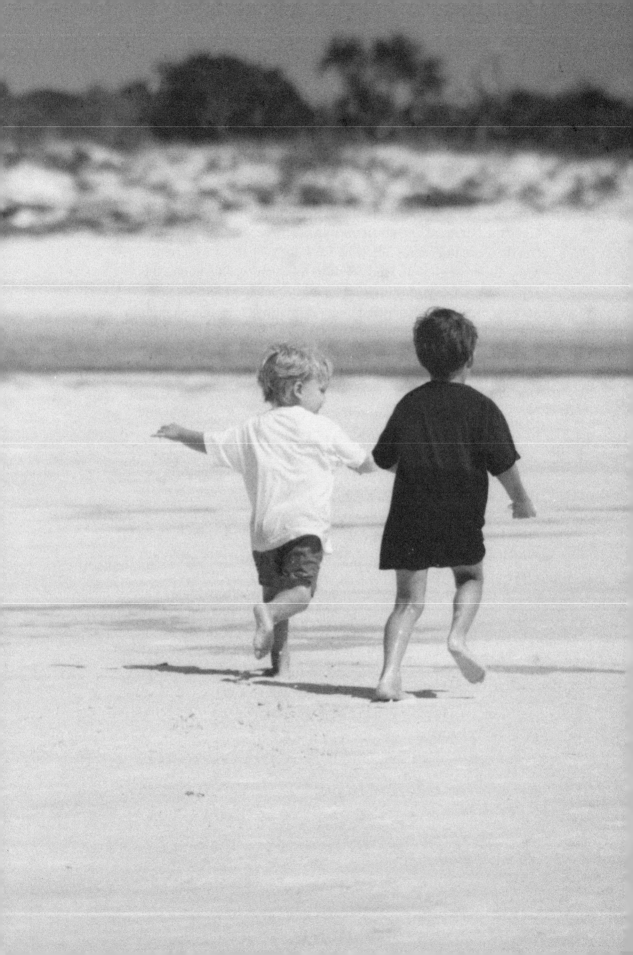

Wrapping the Family in the Quilt

———————————O———————————

National Skills Building Conference
Washington, D.C.
October 10, 1992

The major event in the life of America's AIDS communities in 1992 was the display of the entire AIDS Memorial Quilt in Washington, D.C., during the week of the National Skills Building Conference. When I was invited to address the Conference's luncheon, I felt that—despite unpopular Republican credentials in a politically volatile season—I'd been embraced by the AIDS family.

Mrs. Bush had agreed to visit the Quilt with me during the week, unannounced and unobtrusively—not as a political statement, but as an opportunity to experience its enormity and power. Two mornings in a row we were scheduled to go, and both mornings the massive display was wiped out by rain. We were both disappointed.

I did a national television broadcast that week, and a few other things. But I had my eye on the speech because it was coming at the end of a highly charged, emotional week, at a Saturday noon luncheon attended by leaders from all segments of the AIDS communities. There'd been some talk of splintering and dividing, which I didn't want to encourage. But looking back, what I remember most isn't anything noble or profound; I remember surprising them with a funny line that drew the longest, loudest laugh I'd ever heard from a podium.

I am among the newest members of the HIV/AIDS family which has gathered here this weekend. Last year at this time, I'd just learned I was HIV-positive. I was huddled alone somewhere, hugging myself and my children, racked with anger and fear, uncertain about my future.

This year, I'm here. I've learned to hate the virus, love the family, and be thankful for this reunion and for those of you who have become this family's heroes. I came to Washington, as have many of you, to share the family memorial which is today blanketing the grounds of the Washington Monument. The Quilt reminds us all that ours is a family which is never far from grief.

I think of us less as a movement than as a family. Like other families, we are bound by what's in our blood and in our souls, but we are not all the same—even here, in this room. We are black and white and brown; we are gay and straight, young and old, 999 Democrats and . . . me.

We are not all the same. Not in politics or economic insights. Not in skills or the building of skills. Not in tradition, or in well-being, or in character.

What we share—what binds this family—is a common fear, "the

epidemic," and a common goal, "the cure." Until the day we destroy the virus that now destroys us, we are bound together. We share one overriding passion which dwarfs the importance of our differences and makes us one.

The methods by which we pursue the goal will vary with our gifts. Some stalk the halls of Congress to press for change; others grace the halls of hospitals and hospices, holding the hands of family members no longer able to lead the charge. Some publish. Some march. Some work quietly behind the scenes. Many strategies make strong one family. From the shrill cry of an ACT UP brother to the quiet moaning of a sister whose child will no longer nurse; we are family. From the grief that floods our souls to the comfort we draw from hugs of those who truly understand; we are family.

There are two things I'd like to say today about the role of women in this family. The first is that, as women, we have much to learn from the others.

In America, this virus first took hold within our brothers' gay communities. Like a hurricane of unmatched proportions, this epidemic swept through gay communities leaving behind a diminished and bewildered population. Unlike the outpouring of public sympathy and federal aid which rolled into my home state in the wake of Hurricane Andrew, the response to this epidemic was far too little, far too late, and often far too ugly.

The gay community struggled to come to grips with what was happening to it; graveyards filled faster than research labs. While young men scratched names from address books, wondering what evil lay in wait for them, too many of us listened from a great distance. Not until the virus invaded our own safety did we learn that the experience of the gay community would be our experience as well. Now, with the truth firmly in view, we issue our plea to those who have suffered most: Teach us the lessons you learned without subjecting us to the destruction you endured. Teach us, especially as women, how to bear up with dignity when we are the objects of scorn and abuse. Teach us, especially as women, to unite with all who will support us—lest for the sake of gender we weaken the family whose only strength is found in unity. We have much to learn, as women, from our brothers.

And, as women, we could learn much from each other. We must learn, for example, not to believe our own public images. I've been caricatured as the ex-TV producer and White House staffer who became the model single mom with two preschoolers and one deadly virus who can somehow juggle the household and the children and *The New York Times* editorial board. Does any thoughtful person really believe that in less than a year I came to grips with the crisis of my life, charmed the lions in the Houston den, and went home to make peanut butter sandwiches? You may be told that I'm a mom, an artist, a business partner, a producer, a founder of a national organization, consultant and advisor to a half-dozen others, and an outstanding American in my own right—but who are we kidding?

I'm Mary. And as much as anyone else, I came to Washington this week not to be seen but to grieve; I dreaded the sorrow of this visit. The woman on the world stage *still* has her moments on her bedroom floor hugging herself and her children, sobbing at the thought of losing them. I'm Mary. Pictures on the magazine covers may focus America's attention on the virus; but alone, in the night, wondering where the virus is killing me now, I am no cover girl. I am sad and frightened. . . Mary. On balance, my life is full and satisfying, I am grateful for each day and the spiritual rootedness which I have uncovered. I am not only HIV-positive; I am, most days, positive.

But what I have had the hardest time learning, and still struggle to accept, is that being Mary is enough. That I don't have to do it all and do it perfectly. I'm Mary. That's all I can ever be, and that's all I need to be.

The number of women in the American HIV/AIDS family is rising dramatically, and regrettably. This would be a good time for us to learn from others and from each other that we need not reinvent the organizational wheel. Already we are a genre of literature ("women and AIDS"). Already the cries for research unique to women have been heard, if not acted upon. We must not deny our uniqueness. But we would be wise to seize what we have in common with others in this family and especially to make partners of those who have come before us; they have wisdom our inexperience cannot offer, and they have proven a courage which we have not yet demonstrated on our own. In the wake of discovering that we are HIV-positive women, we must not let ourselves be separated from women in general—we are not less women because we are HIV-positive.

And, whoever you are, male or female, it is enough. Do what you do best, and stop. If you can teach, teach; if you can write laws, or songs, or letters to the editor, write. March if you can. Heal if you can. Pray if you can. If knowing the agony of this disease, all you can do is grieve, then grieve. Stand in public and sob until someone asks you why and tell them.

As women—and as men—we have much to learn from each other. And that's my first point. My second is this: Women already have a place in this family.

We do not need to bang on doors that are not closed and knock down walls of our own making. In this family's history, from the beginning, women have been seated at the table with men. Some of us suffered the virus. Many of us did not and we were there anyway.

June Osborn[1] was there early on, burning midnight hours in laboratories and living rooms, issuing warning cries in classrooms

[1]Dr. June Osborn, M.D.—Chairwoman of the U.S. National Commission on AIDS, Dean and Professor, School of Public Health at the University of Michigan.

and in cloakrooms. Sandra McDonald[2] was there, reaching up, reaching out, and teaching others to reach with her. Paula Van Ness[3] was there. Mathilde Krim[4] was there. Sally Fisher[5] was there. And a hundred more in this room today, unnoticed and unnamed, you were there.

And now come we, the much-heralded late arrivals. Our role—*my* role—in this family is not first to lead, but to serve. If there are barriers to our service within this family, I have not found them. What's lacking isn't volunteers for leadership, but for service.

The place of women in American history has not always been recognized. But yesterday morning I stood on the platform preparing to read names, waiting for the Quilt to be unfurled, knowing that the history of American women would be rolled out before me.

Because, more than a century ago, before radios and telephones and fax machines; before Dorthea Dix humanized mental health and *Uncle Tom's Cabin* shook the morality from slavery; before many American women had learned to read, there was the quilting bee, the weekly community of women. They came together bearing rags and needles and thread and courage. They sewed, they talked, they survived.

It was over the quilt that they discovered each other and them-

---

[2]Sandra McDonald—President and Founder of OUTREACH, Inc., the first minority AIDS agency established in the State of Georgia (perhaps one of the oldest in the South).

[3]Paula Van Ness—Executive Director of the National Community AIDS Partnership (NCAP).

[4]Dr. Mathilde Krim, Ph.D.—Founding Co-Chairman of the Board of the American Foundation for AIDS Research (AmFAR). Academic appointment to Columbia University's School of Public Health as Adjunct Professor of Public Health.

[5]Sally Fisher—Founder of Northern Lights in Los Angeles, California, author of *Life Mastery*, leader of "Taking Care" workshops for care providers, and Program Director of The Resources for Experimental AIDS Therapies (T.R.E.A.T.) in Santa Fe, New Mexico.

selves. Here they broke the silence. Here they told the secrets of childbearing and women's health. Here they offered cures and sympathy, recipes and warnings. As needles traced intricate patterns in an uniquely feminine art form, they kept alive their mothers' tradition and their daughters' hope.

Week after week, into the quilt, they stitched the family's memories. In the blue gingham sewn by aging hands lived the memories of a Saturday dance. In the white cotton was an infant's cry; in the red patchwork, the smell of a grandfather's pipe. They were all there, the family members, every one of them remembered by a patch.

When the cold winter winds whistled across the prairie, it was the quilt that warmed the children. When the fevers broke out and bodies broke down, a mother's sleepless hands lifted both her prayer and her quilt a little higher. When the bride and groom found the magic of their bed, there was the quilt. And when, no longer newlyweds, they carried their first child to the grave, they laid her down to rest in the quilt.

When, a century later, some San Francisco friends decided that each name of lost loved ones should be captured on a Quilt, the history of women was woven into the history of AIDS in America.

Therefore, we women need not fight to find our place. It has been given to us. We need only be true to who we are, women; to do what women have done through the centuries: Wrap the family in the Quilt. If women can contribute such strength of unity, then they will have done a great deal.

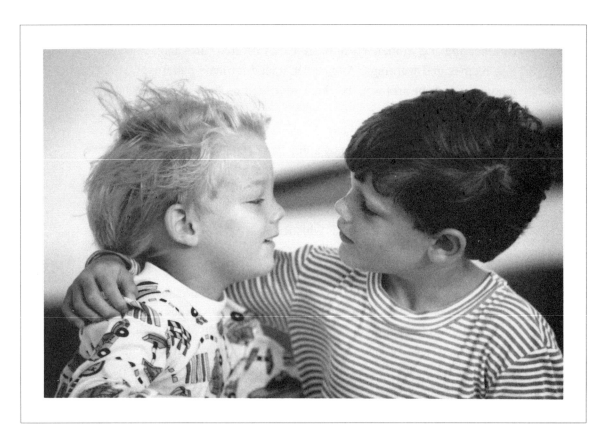

A Call to Partnership

———————— Ө ————————

Community Leader Forum
Greensboro, North Carolina
October 13, 1992

The morning after I'd given the Quilt speech I flew to Charlotte, North Carolina, to begin a three-day regional tour of speeches and events.

We'd selected North Carolina, based on advice from AIDS leaders there, as a place where we might help change community attitudes toward the disease and those who suffer from it. We thought that, especially in conservative communities, my Republican credentials might help challenge misperceptions about the epidemic.

On Sunday (October 11) I spoke at worship services in Charlotte and Concord. Monday was a news conference, community events, more interviews, and an ecumenical memorial service for those who'd lost loved ones to AIDS. By Tuesday we were in Greensboro, where an audience of several hundred community leaders had been gathered.

Under ordinary circumstances, I'd have welcomed this moment. But circumstances weren't ordinary. I was exhausted from the pace we'd set. I'd been traveling, away from home and children for more than a week. And, worst, it was October 13— Max's fifth birthday—and I had several speeches to finish before I could head home.

I hope you'll forgive me, but I have a personal favor to ask before I begin. You may have noticed that I'm carrying the curse of our modern existence, a cellular phone. I have my son Max on the phone, and this is Max's fifth birthday. He is not overjoyed at the fact that his mom isn't there this morning, so I just explained that I had a whole chorus of people with me who'd be delighted to sing "Happy Birthday" to him over the telephone. So, if you'd like to help me rescue a relationship which has five years of important history, I'd be grateful if someone would hit the right pitch and start singing to Max.

. . .Thanks!

I'm frequently asked what I've told my children about the fact that I am HIV-positive. The truth is, I've said very little because they're so young. Max turns five today and Zachary turns three on Saturday. Like all preschoolers, they take their Mom for granted. And since I'm as healthy as any other Mom, they have no cause to wonder or ask hard questions.

Besides, life at our house is very ordinary. The virus I contracted in my marriage can be transmitted sexually or through direct, blood-to-blood contact: transfusions, needle-exchanges, and so forth. But you can't transmit it by hugs or kisses or loving each other. My kids still climb into mom's bed, which somehow sleeps better, and eat the food off my plate which must taste better.

Some people are surprised to know how ordinary our lives are. Perhaps they do not know that the human immunodeficiency virus—HIV—

destroys the body's immune system very slowly, usually over a period of a decade or more. AIDS is the name given to late-stage HIV infection; nothing new has happened, really, it's just that the virus has weakened the body so other killers can come by and finish the job. People don't die of AIDS; they ordinarily die of pneumonia or cancer or other infections.

These are simple facts, but they're important if we're ever going to make sense out of the following five points:

First, HIV-positive people aren't ordinarily included in epidemic numbers. When you hear "AIDS statistics," you need to multiply by up to ten times that number to estimate the number of infected—HIV-positive—people. This confusion has resulted in a false sense of safety for the public. Good people, seeing low numbers, have asked: "Why so much attention to this one illness?"

Point two: The problem is, everyone who is HIV-positive will develop AIDS, and one-and-a-half or two million Americans are already HIV-positive. I'm one of them and you know others (Magic Johnson, for example). If the Americans now infected are to survive, a "cure on the order of a miracle" would be needed immediately. Even if we stopped the *spread* of the epidemic today, which we can't, perhaps two million Americans—most at ages typically associated with the pink of health—will flood the healthcare system with AIDS.

Third, worldwide estimates range from 40 to 110 million HIV cases within the coming two decades. The numbers are staggering, especially when you take them one at a time, which is how HIV takes us. This is not only an epidemic: It's an epidemic of unimagined proportions.

Fourth, the rate of growth is not a straight line; it's an upward curve. The virus was first identified and named in 1981. It took ten years for America to log its first 100,000 deaths attributed to AIDS. It will take less than two years for the second 100,000 deaths because the epidemic grows exponentially. One HIV-positive person can infect a dozen others. Symptoms may not develop for a decade, so entire networks may be infected before anyone is aware of the crisis. That's why we so often speak of the urgent need for awareness.

Point five: If you think this is someone else's disease, you're out-of-date. I thought that myself until last summer, when a phone call changed my life. It's sheer historical coincidence that, in America, this disease first appeared in gay communities. Worldwide, that's not true. And today, in America, that's not true. The fastest growing HIV-positive populations in the U.S. are women, children and young adults. This year new infections will be reported in nearly equal numbers between women and men.

So if you think your family and your community are immune for some reason, think again. Five years ago, one out of every twenty Americans knew personally someone who was HIV-positive; today, it is one out of every four; in three years, the ratio will be a perfect one-to-one.

That is why we need partnerships, and need them urgently. We need research which has been planned but not initiated, because there are no funding partners. We need partnerships between the public and private sectors, partnerships to be forged by thoughtful leaders—like you. We need bold leadership from journalists and broadcasters, educators and opinion shapers—leadership based on fact, not fiction; on current knowledge, not historic myths. You do not need to leave your field of service to be enlisted as a partner in this war; we need you where you are, using the truth to its best advantage.

We need partnerships to fight a virus that breaks down the body. But we also need partnerships to heal the wounds which have resulted from breakdowns in your communities. Because more than any other disease in the history of America, the story of HIV and AIDS has been told with prejudice, punctuated by ignorance, and marred by stigma and shame.

You and I, together, cannot stop the breakdown of my immune system. Not knowing what we know today. But together, with each other, we have the power to halt the breakdowns that have accompanied this epidemic. We have learned enough. We have been taught that we are not yet a people immune to prejudice and hatred. Those who contracted the fatal virus often died twice: first, we destroyed their self-image, their hope, their dignity—we assigned them to a category of shame. Then we left them to the virus which finished the job. We have sometimes preferred silence over courage; we have tolerated discrimination when we could have insisted on compassion.

Perhaps we cannot defeat the virus. But we can challenge the legacy of meanness, we can take on the brutality of judgment, and we can reject the call to ignorance—if we choose.

We need partners, men and women willing to prove within their communities that personal character is more important than crude popularity. We need some partners with courage.

We need partners who, hearing the whispers of discrimination in the workplace, will say "no" to those who hate; partners who, seeing the need for a place to die in dignity, will say "yes" to those who suffer. We need partners unwilling to throw the first stone and eager to take up the cause of those too weakened, too frightened, and too sick to take it up themselves. We need partners with integrity.

You sang "Happy Birthday" to one of my sons this morning. I need not be maudlin for you to understand that, of course, I would like to see their high school graduation, their wives, their children. Of course I would. But I am powerless to add one day to my life, and so are you.

But we could forge a partnership to change the environment in which we live every day God gives us. As partners, we could call for a world marked by better justice, so that when they cross the stage to get their diplomas they do not suffer stigma on my account. We could work for communities of acceptance, so that when I am no longer able to bear them up or carry them through, others will fill the void I did not mean to create. We could search for leaders who will not wait for the cause to become popular.

We will know our partners when we see them, and they will know themselves. They are the ones who, when they truly see the crisis at our door, will say to themselves: "If not me, who? If not now, when?"

Do not leave this place today without committing yourself to such a partnership. You need not do it for me; I'm flying home to a birthday boy. Do it for yourself, your community, your children.

There's no better gift you could give, whether or not it is a birthday.

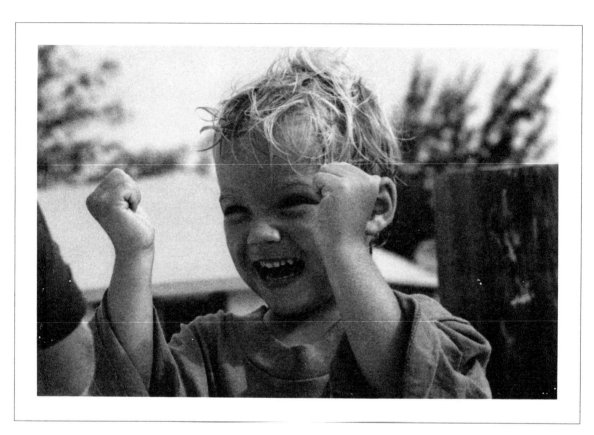

Keeping Hope Alive

———————o———————

Dana-Farber Cancer Institute Annual Meeting
Boston
October 25, 1992

Dr. William Haseltine of the Dana-Farber Cancer Institute at Harvard University is well-known in AIDS communities. Critical research being completed by him and the Institute's staff is one of our few lines to encouragement that there may, someday, be a cure. I was happy to accept his invitation to speak at the Institute's annual meeting—and to explain, firsthand, the urgency of his work.

What I did not know is that Dr. Haseltine would, just before I spoke, provide dazzlingly depressing statistics. He doubted that anyone infected today would ever be cured based on the pace of research and discoveries. What's more, while Americans have not yet accepted the fact that this epidemic will surely kill tens of millions, Haseltine thought it was time "we look toward the year 2020 when we will count deaths due to AIDS in the billions."

When he had finished his litany of doom, he warmly introduced me and my topic: hope.

The Dana-Farber Cancer Institute's work in HIV/AIDS research is a pioneer task on a troubled frontier. At the one extreme are reputable scientists who fear that HIV will baffle researchers for decades to come. Such reports open the floodgates of terror for the million-and-a-half Americans already infected. At the other extreme are persistent rumors of cures already known but hidden, and vaccines invented but not announced.

And the link between cancer research and AIDS research is more than accidental. HIV weakens us by destroying our immune systems so other causes, notably cancer, can kill us. Since the earliest days of the epidemic, improved knowledge about cancer treatment has saved the lives of persons with AIDS. Research in each area serves interests in the other.

You know, of course, that I am not here today because of my scientific exploits. I am here to remind you that there is a direct correlation between scientific research and human hope. In some sense, I am not only your speaker but your example of how these come together.

For some, research is a matter of refined technology; for others of us, it is the substance of human hope. To staff here, it is career; to me, it is promise. It's the key to my parents' comfort, my sisters' encouragement, my brother's joy. And it's the avenue by which I will travel far into my children's future.

The man who devotes his life to research is drawn back to the laboratory in the wee hours of the night; he's driven to follow one obtuse clue, as surely as I am drawn back to my children's bedrooms for one last stroke of their cheeks, and one final prayer. What drives his research is hope; what sustains my hope is his research.

Science imposes boundaries on research. At the same moment our knowledge opens new vistas, our ignorance draws the horizon beyond which we cannot go. My gratitude to you—and the gratitude of the entire HIV/AIDS community—is driven by the certainty that many of you are pushing back those limits. You are the ones who will one day crack open the door behind which lurks the discovery that would justify my family's hope.

With research, science imposes the limits. But with hope, we create our own boundaries.

Listen to the boots of goosestepping soldiers marching into Paris and Amsterdam, and you hear the sound that crushed hope for a generation. Look into the eyes of an African mother holding the emaciated body of her child, and you see a vacant stare where hope was once alive.

Hope thrives where there is compassion. But the story of HIV/AIDS in America is a history in which compassion has played far too small a role. In the earliest days—when most Americans believed this was a virus contained within the gay communities—for every voice of sympathy there was a chorus of moral indignation. The illness itself inherited a legacy of bigotry. Those with HIV soon discovered that to admit their diagnoses was to proclaim oneself a modern-day leper. HIV exposed those who carried it not only to the physical challenge of a lifetime, but also to the social, psychological and spiritual trauma of one who is considered "unclean." Physicians refused treatment; dentists turned down patients. Hospitals wrote "HIV-positive" on doors and patient name tags. Schools barred children from admission. While young men grew weak and died, families turned away.

My journey as a spokesperson for the cause has been easy by comparison to what was suffered by the pioneers a decade ago. The environment had already begun to change when I arrived. Our national response gained momentum when we learned that this virus could not be, and had not been, contained to the gay community. When young Ryan White grew ill, that's when sympathy grew louder. When the blood supply which any of us might need was tainted, then we responded. This history suggests, of course, that it was not compassion but merely self-interest that fueled our increased national concern. While I welcome the new concern, it is important that we not confuse it with compassion.

Today, an epidemic of unmatched and unimaginable proportions is sweeping our nation. It's true that we have lacked political consensus. And it's true that we have lacked adequate funding. But above all, what we have lacked is pure compassion. The families of those infected have listened to a decade of debate about the morality of their dying loved ones. In the place of official concern they have weathered years of indifference. We must learn again, as history has too often taught us, that when compassion is unseen, hope fades. And as hope shrivels, anger mounts.

We may sometimes think of science and research as abstract skills practiced in hermetically sealed environments. But it isn't so. Dana-Farber Institute lives and breathes in an atmosphere of social agony regarding AIDS. And that is why I salute the Institute and those who support it today. Because you have gone forward with commitment, you have mounted a serious offensive against a brutal enemy. You have demonstrated through policies and programs that compassion is more than a sympathetic word: It is brave action and hard work.

Not all in the HIV/AIDS community will trust you; not all will support me. But what matters is that we act wisely—that we do what we do best, and do it with wisdom. If you have time to donate, give it freely. If you have the gifts of science and administration, put them to work here. If you can teach, teach understanding. If you can write, write about justice. In it all, compose a life of compassion. But do not lose sight of the history behind us or the agony around us.

If we can maintain perspective then, when we hear the shrill protests of those who have grown hopelessly angry, we will recall the decade of indifference that has driven out their hope. We will respond with wisdom, not with anger.

When we see the rage of those who have buried too many friends, lost too many loved ones, heard too many excuses—we will know that they have suffered enough. We will welcome those who protest what others of us have too easily, too silently, and too long accepted.

And we will, day by day, do what we do best. Those of you who labor here—in research and administration, in education and development—do what you do best, because it is a most critical task. You are the magnet which attracts our hope. If not for my sake, then for the sake of my children, you must not give up the search. Demand that we provide the resources you need; shout from the rooftops if more is required. Be relentless in your science and brave in your policies. If it were not life-and-death, I would not ask that you exhaust yourselves and all you have for this mission. But it is. And so I ask you to give it all you have, knowing that you are surrounded by our prayers both day and night.

Some of you have lost loved ones. You have a special role among us, because you can remind us of our focus. I do not need to tell you what wakes me in the night. You know how and why I cling to my children. You know firsthand the numbing grief that breaks over us like waves. You remember the somber-faced surgeons who said they'd done the best they could. You recall the long days and even longer nights in which courage failed you and all you had left was tears. You understand the seething rage that makes you shake your fist at God. This agony—this cutting edge of cruel despair—has made you rich in understanding.

Therefore, all of you here today, the family of the Dana-Farber Institute, are a reason for hope. My children and I, and all of us within the HIV/AIDS family, are in your debt. Since we are unable to repay you, we thank you—and we ask that you go forward with courage and with compassion. Without courage, we would give up the battle. Without compassion, the battle has no purpose.

But armed with both courage and compassion, even this—the most stubborn and deadly of viruses—cannot defeat us. We can keep hope alive. And I would like to do that with you. I would like to be your colleague, going into God's future beside you, sharing the task, pursuing the hope, and celebrating the compassion which marks us all.

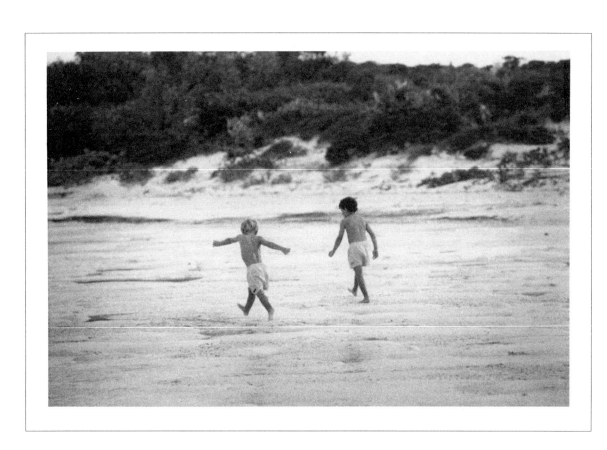

Coming Home with Joy

———————————— o ————————————

Walk for Life
West Palm Beach, Florida
November 1, 1992

AIDS organizations across America have raised both funds and consciousness through community AIDS walks in recent years. In early October I'd spoken at the kickoff for such a walk in Santa Fe, New Mexico, where my friend Sally Fisher had opened my eyes and my heart to the reality of my own virus a year earlier.

My brief remarks at the West Palm Beach walk, held just a few miles from where I then lived, were similar to what I'd said in Santa Fe. What was different wasn't the speech, but the friends: Joy Anderson and Joy Prouty. Anderson and I are godmothers for each other's children. She's been a source of love and encouragement—and last-minute childcare—on countless occasions.

And then there is Joy Prouty. Despite her full-time career and her international travel schedule, she always has time for me. During the first days following my diagnosis when I couldn't sleep—when I would sit, arms wrapped around my knees, and shake—Joy Prouty would sit with me, talking. When I decided to tell my story publicly, she was there at midnight, standing by the fax machine as newspaper copy from Detroit rolled onto my study floor.

This little speech was, in fact, less about a walk than about love.

A year ago, my incredible friend Joy Prouty wanted me to come walk with you. I'd recently discovered that I was HIV-positive. I'd told my family and close friends, but I hadn't really gotten through the process of explaining it to myself. I was confused and angry and, especially, I was frightened.

I told Joy I'd go with her. But when that Sunday morning dawned a year ago, I could not come. I stayed home and held my children. I rocked and I wondered. . .and I cried that day. And Joy Prouty said it was okay, we'd go another time.

This is "another time," Joy. I'm here to walk. And I've brought not one Joy, but two: Joy Prouty, and Joy Anderson, two very special friends. I am here in large measure because of you, the people who are here with me. My two Joys have lifted me over mountains and carried me over deserts in the past year. I was not summoned to this walk, I was hugged into it.

Today, I am here—not only able to walk, but eager. Because of you, I'm here today, stumbling less and celebrating more. Oh, I hate the virus and I'll never welcome AIDS. But with the challenge has come meaning which, over time, squeezes out anger.

With the pain have come occasions to demonstrate for my children, and even for myself, that courage taken in small doses can do a great deal.

The number of ways people fight AIDS is amazing. Some teach children how to protect themselves from the epidemic; some show children how to live with it. Some draft laws or challenge policy makers. Some raise funds, others raise awareness. They care for the sick, comfort the orphans, and refuse to be silenced in their demands for action. I've seen them in hospitals and hospices, from Amsterdam to Arizona, making their contribution in the fight. Today, you and I will contribute—by walking.

Walking is an important symbol in this fight. It's an act of confidence, demonstrating a great exodus from the fear and ignorance, the suspicion and prejudice which have attacked the AIDS community in the past. We will march toward justice and compassion and hope, knowing that where we find these, there we will find healing.

Walking is an act of solidarity. We'll walk today in a great company made up not only of the hundreds who are here, but also the millions who are members of the worldwide HIV/AIDS family. We walk with famous friends: Elizabeth and Bob and Ryan and Arthur, and my friend Magic who not only walks, he runs, he shoots, he makes me laugh.

And walking is an expression of our hope. Where hope dies, so does humanity—therefore, to walk for life *is* to walk for hope. Those of you who have already lost a loved one, take comfort: Whether or not you can see them this afternoon, or feel the touch of their hand—as we walk together, we walk again with them. Those of you who are HIV-positive, look about you and take strength: These are the people who will bear us up when it is hard to stand on our own. For those who have come uncertain of why you are here, frightened, fearful, even angry: Welcome. You've come as *I* was *un*able to come a year ago: Welcome to our family. Welcome home.

So we will walk today. Don't go too fast or I won't be able to keep up! But go with joy: Hug a friend and hoist a child up on your shoulders; skip and dance and laugh along the way. Make of this walk a giant drama whose plot is life over death. In fact, it's a love story: As Joy, and Joy, and others have loved me out of a shell of self-pity and into the sunlight of hope, we'll love into our midst all who see us today.

Because the virus cannot destroy us, let us walk. In wheelchairs and Reeboks, let us walk. In laughter and longing, through memories and neighborhoods; with joy in the noisy company and hope in the quiet of our souls—let us walk!

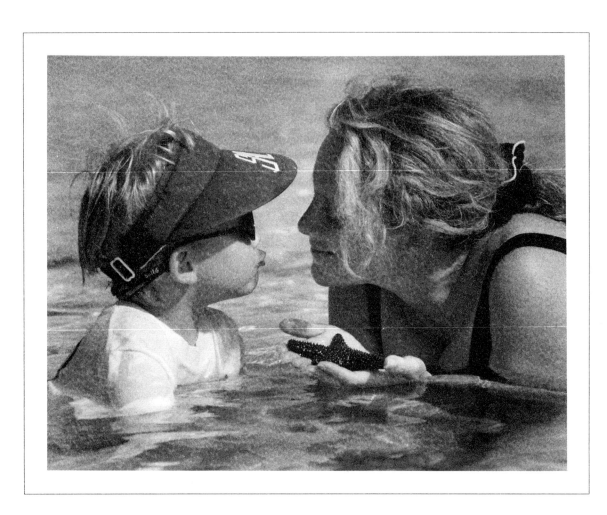

The Courage to Be Compassionate

————————o————————

Planned Parenthood
Palm Beach, Florida
November 5, 1992

I'd been in North Carolina for Max's birthday, and I was in Florida for my mother's. She was in Detroit, and one of her Palm Beach friends, Ann Appleman, had asked that I speak to a group of Planned Parenthood supporters and staff in a community where poverty is often discussed but rarely experienced.

The meeting was held in a spacious, sunlit home, attended by women who thought, as I once had, that AIDS is a threat to others but not to themselves. Many were women of wealth and influence, and I was eager to increase their support for local AIDS organizations.

But the speech itself was not really about AIDS. It was about us and our values, our attitudes, our beliefs about community, our concern to set new models for our children. AIDS demands that, as parents and community leaders, we set a moral course. In fact, it demands compassion—which, because it is more than niceness, may require of us a good deal of courage.

I am genuinely honored to be here. If I were a better daughter, I would be attending my mother's birthday party in Detroit. Well, I've already given my mother 44 years, so I figured I owed Ann Appleman an afternoon. I have a suggestion for you, Ann, when you get home, call my mother. I'd start by saying Happy Birthday.

I regard any invitation from Planned Parenthood to be a personal tribute. Among volunteer organizations serving our communities and our nation, none has retained a more dignified presence under greater scrutiny than Planned Parenthood. Despite great misunderstanding and considerable hostility, Planned Parenthood has been a model of grace under pressure, meeting a need unmet—and, sadly, unattempted—in other quarters. So I am honored that you would invite me to be your guest today.

But I am not only honored. I am also concerned—concerned that the fight against HIV/AIDS in America continues to garner the full support of organizations like Planned Parenthood. Some of you here today may be new to the struggle with HIV/AIDS. I have only a year's experience of intense involvement myself. Some of you are already veterans in this battle. You are Planned Parenthood educators and social workers who joined the ranks of those struggling against the most extensive, deadliest epidemic in history. You have committed not only your careers, but your lives, to the effort. You are heroes in my eyes.

But, whatever brought you here this afternoon, each of you is critical to the task at hand. As parents and partners, as volunteers and role models, as community leaders and family members, each of you has a role which only you can play in this drama. So I need to speak personally to each of you.

It could be argued that government has not done enough; I think it has not. It could be argued that the temple and church have not led an adequate moral response; I think that's largely true. We could argue about media who have been content with ignorance and health professionals who have distanced themselves from this crisis. We could argue long and hard. But listen: We don't really have time to argue long and hard. We don't have time to argue at all. Since we came into this home, another half-dozen Americans have contracted HIV and started down the road to AIDS. We need action and we need it now.

And here is my appeal to you: Whatever it is that you do best, bring that gift to the party. Do what you do best in the fight against HIV/AIDS.

If you are a parent, learn the facts and have the courage to open a conversation with your children. Tell your children that you love them and want them to live long, healthy lives—and then prove you told them the truth by *helping* them live long, healthy lives: Explain the facts about HIV and AIDS. If someone told me they loved me but withheld the information which would spare my life, what kind of love would that be?

If you live in a home or work in a context where religious and moral values are important, I urge you to hold them high. Have the courage to teach others about grace, even when it is tempting to engage in less worthy judgmentalism. Explain our need to behave justly toward others, and to fill our lives with compassion, so that life takes on the character of service which gives it meaning.

And I introduce those two concepts—justice and compassion—because of the history of HIV/AIDS in America. The record which will be written of the first ten years of this epidemic is one of ignorance, prejudice, and shame. Persons on deathbeds have been told that they deserve their condition, that it is God's sentence on their behaviors—

as if our behaviors, whatever they may be, will somehow cost or fetch us a special spot in God's eyes. Children have been barred from admission to schools and, perhaps more painfully, from play with other children. Public policy and private practice have both been forged from pure ignorance and ugly prejudice. Adults have wallowed contentedly in pools of mythology about this illness, unwilling to ask direct questions or hear honest answers. And so we have given the virus a nearly perfect culture in which to grow.

In the face of that history, I appeal to you to take courage and begin modelling compassion. If we are compassionate, we will not let children pass through our lives too ignorant to protect their own. If we are compassionate, we will not teach others—by our behaviors—to practice discrimination and foster ignorance. If we are compassionate, we will not go quietly into the night while others die by the score; we will raise first our consciousness, and then our voices, in the campaign against this killer.

I know that it takes courage to step forward when a cause is sometimes unpopular and positions are easily misunderstood. Believe me, I know. I know both from struggling to find the courage myself and from seeing it in others. When speaking out seemed the hardest thing to do, when my parents struggled to come to grips with this crisis, those are the times our friend, Ann Appleman, proved her courage with compassion. Because, without courage, there can be no compassion. Courage requires that we place others ahead of ourselves, and compassion provides the motivation.

The most powerful influences in my own life were not distant heroes brought to me on the silver screen or television tube. They were real-life people of flesh-and-blood. My parents. A teacher. A friend and a mentor. They were common people, by and large; common people marked by uncommon grace. They knew justice firsthand and lived lives overflowing with decency and compassion.

In my own attempts at imitation, however feeble and flawed, they became the model of my own future.

In the lives of your community, your workplace, your family, you are those people. You are the models that will be imitated when your children talk and your neighbors vote, when policy is considered and prejudice is tried out. You are the models that will be copied time and time again. If you demand justice, if you abhor stigma, if you reject judgmentalism and embrace dignity, so will others around you.

Perhaps some of you know this fable:

Once upon a time there was a little old man. His eyes blinked and his hands trembled; when he ate he clattered the silverware distressingly, missed his mouth with the spoon as often as not, and dribbled a bit of his food on the tablecloth.

Now he lived with his married son, having nowhere else to live, and his son's wife was a modern young woman who knew that in-laws should not be tolerated in a woman's home.

"I can't have this," she said. "It interferes with a woman's right to happiness."

So she and her husband took the little old man gently but firmly by the arm and led him to the corner of the kitchen. There they set him on a stool and gave him his food, what there was of it, in an earthenware bowl. From then on he always ate in the corner, blinking at the table with wistful eyes.

One day his hands trembled rather more than usual, and the earthenware bowl fell and broke.

"If you are a pig," said the daughter-in-law, "you must eat out of a trough." So they made him a little wooden trough, and he got his meals in that.

These people had a four-year-old son of whom they were very fond. One suppertime the young man noticed his boy playing intently with some bits of wood and asked what he was doing.

"I'm making a trough," he said, smiling up for approval, "to feed you and Mama out of when I get big."

Whatever else we are doing in our lives, we are inevitably—because others are watching—teaching our own values to those who are most vulnerable. If we value courage, we will show it; if we value compassion, we will have it.

If we cannot grasp a cure, we can seize the suffering which is within our power to relieve. We can oppose injustice and encourage compassion; we can embrace those who suffer and defend their cause.

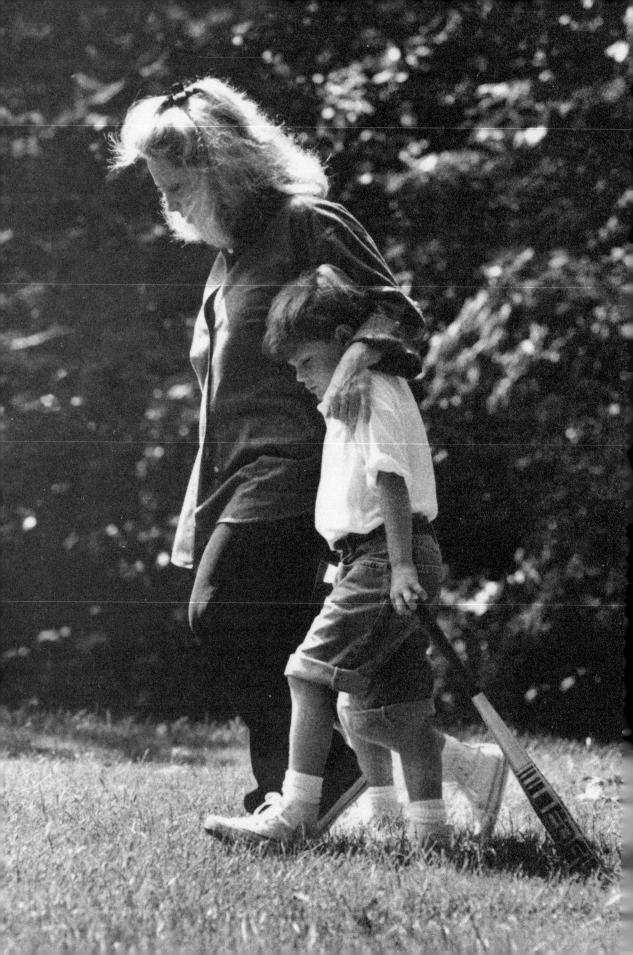

When Grief Meets Grace

———————o———————

Church of the Valley
Van Nuys, California
November 8, 1992

Spirituality gives us depth. It's where we sink our roots so we can grow. It's what enables us to capture and hold a broad, clear picture of reality—where we can see that we are called to a higher purpose than self-service and self-satisfaction.

America's organized religious communities—the corner church and neighborhood temple—have rejected AIDS patients at least as often as they have accepted them. Many of the rejections have been especially shameful, done as they were in the name of God.

I'm convinced we'll win the war against this epidemic only when religious communities go to the front of the battle. I've

been eager to call them into service through speeches and even,
as in this instance, through an occasional sermon.

    This sermon was based on two biblical texts: from the Old
Testament, II Samuel 18:24-33 (the story of King David's grief
at the death of his son Absalom) and, from the New Testament,
Hebrews 11:32-12:2 (where early martyrs, "of whom the
world is not worthy," were encouraged to keep the faith).

Growing up in a Jewish home near Detroit, my parents encouraged me to adopt lofty goals. Preaching sermons in Christian congregations was not one of them.

My mother, whose spiritual journey has helped shape my own, said she would come with me this morning—and she has. Like most grown daughters, I've been waiting forty-some years to give *her* a sermon . . . so that alone makes this worthwhile.

Actually, I've never doubted the worthwhileness of worship. I *did* doubt, at least briefly, my qualifications for this assignment. But someone close to me and close to your tradition said, "Well, Mary, if they'd invited Jesus to preach, they'd have gotten someone just like you: A spokesperson for a misunderstood cause, raised in a good Jewish family, with strong Christian sympathies." I like being in that company, and in yours, so I'm pleased to be here.

A little more than a year ago I discovered I am HIV-positive, that I'm traveling at an uncertain pace toward AIDS. Coming to grips with our own mortality is a perspective-giving moment. In my own case, the perspective is largely spiritual. It's rooted in the biblical perspective that human history is an unfolding drama which swings between aching grief and stunning grace. Grief and grace—like magnetic poles, pulsating throughout our lives, tugging us back and forth from cradle to grave.

Most of us would gladly take a pass on grief; but we cannot. Unavoidably, inevitably, the moments come when we are drenched in grief. The parent who has been our strength is suddenly childlike, dying; the relationship that we trusted is shattered by deceit; a doctor announces test results that weaken our knees. Barely able to breathe or see, we are wrenched away from public headlines and public performance; we are staggered, dropped to our knees, face-to-face with the reality of grief. We cannot grow beyond it—no matter who we are or what we have. Even King David could only struggle up a stairway to sob alone: "O my son Absalom. . .my son, my son Absalom! If only I had died instead of you—O Absalom, my son, my son. . . ."

Adults forget how early grief invades our lives. We forget the terror of being embarrassed by a teacher who may not like us, the brutality of a playground where we are alone, the life-ending agony of being rejected for dropping a fly ball or wearing the wrong skirt. I tell you: Grief comes early and stays late in life.

But grief is only one pole. Grace is the other, and it is the one that surprises us most. We leave the mortuary feeling empty and wasted; a week or two later, we notice the gentle curve of a rainbow and feel a strange peace. A friend we admire at school tells us we are her hero. We feel the delicious joy of a child's morning hug after we spent a sleepless night. We hear the quiet whisper of "I love you," coming out of the darkness from someone we thought was sleeping. We are surprised by grace.

The turns between grief and grace are sometimes sudden in our lives, as they are in Scripture. The opening of Psalm 22, "My God, my God, why have you forsaken me?" is still echoing when we hear the next Psalm begin: "The Lord is my shepherd . . . I shall not want (Psalm 23)."

When I was a little girl, my grandmother taught me to cross-stitch; still hanging on my wall is my first effort: the 23rd Psalm. It was there a year ago when I heard myself gasping, "My God, my God, why. . . ?"

Since the beginning of the HIV/AIDS epidemic, grief has been the constant companion of those infected and most affected by the virus. Grace has not been absent, but grief has clearly dominated.

We often think of grief as a brief stage of mourning. But living with HIV extends the duration of grief to the length of a lifetime. Most of us infected with HIV are healthy. So we live, infected, wondering what will give in first, and last; unsure what promise to make to our children, or ourselves; wondering when the distant bell will suddenly toll more closely. We do not so much recover from this grief as learn to live with it. It is an unhappy albatross hung about the necks of nearly two million Americans.

Because the epidemic first surfaced in America within gay communities, this grief has been compounded. Old patterns of discrimination came to life with new brutality. Traditional sources of comfort—the home and the church—became, instead, tribunals of judgment. Parents rejected children. Young men, untrained in nursing skills, cared first for dying friends and then died themselves, alone—because the homes from which they had come were now closed to them. Voices rang out from pulpits saying the virus was God's idea, speculating that HIV was divine retribution. Intimate messages of rejection were matched by public policies of indifference. Not until the virus jumped all social fences, putting all of us at risk, did the nation respond. Our response was fueled by self-interest more than compassion. In the end, the HIV/AIDS community was blanketed with a grief too deep for consolation.

For the HIV/AIDS community in America, the voice of God heard from communities of faith has been terribly muted. Temples should have raised high the roofbeams to bring them in; churches should have shouted messages of grace from the rooftop. But what most members of the HIV/AIDS family have heard is whispers about their morality and the hope that—like modern-day lepers—they will not get too close. And so the peculiar grief has grown, fed by shame and ignorance, stigma and rejection.

If you take the great sweep of redemptive history as told in the Bible, it has a simple theme: The antidote to our grief is God's grace. When we cannot save ourselves, God redeems us. When we are beyond hope, he rescues us. In our deaths he gives us new life. In our agony, he touches us with comfort.

To suggest that the God of Scripture hurls HIV and AIDS at his children is profanity. To imagine that some of us are more worthy of grace than others is hypocrisy. There is nothing in ourselves that earns grace, else it is not grace at all. Because grace is love *undeserved*. Grace is the rescue we can't perform, the comfort we can't grasp. And the good news—the "gospel"—is this: Trapped in our grief, God comes in grace to set us free.

This is grace: When your child tries and fails, and ruins your family name; when he tells you secrets you hope the neighbors never uncover; when he says, "I've been arrested," when she blurts out, "I had an abortion," when full of fear they, trembling, stammer, "I wanted to die. . . ." When at that moment neither pride nor reputation slow you down on your rush to lift them up, cradle them in your arms, kiss their tears and tell them you love them—this is love undeserved. Grace.

This is grace: The high school senior was undergoing cancer therapy. On top of the crushing fear and daily nausea, he suffered the added indignity of losing all his hair. Still, when the day came that the therapy ended, he headed back for school. When he walked through the door that first morning, there were all of his friends with shining bald heads. They had, every one of them, shaved their scalps clean. They could not take his cancer, but they could relieve his shame. And so, with a special and—as always!—surprising grace, they welcomed him with laughter and with baldness.

You who are here, in God's house, surely, you have been surprised by grace in your own lives. All that I ask of you—perhaps all that God asks of you—is that you show it to others.

The HIV-positive man in Studio City whose family has told him not to come home; surprise him with grace, if you can. The mother with AIDS in downtown Los Angeles who cannot imagine how her children will survive as orphans; become grace in her life. The infant in the nearby hospital wrapped in tubes and rarely held; the person sitting here this morning, shivering in fear at the thought of being uncovered—these are God's children waiting for grace from you.

What's needed today is more heroes like those described in the letter written to the Jewish-Christian community, the chapter from Hebrews read earlier. Rome occupied Israel and brought with its occupation adoration for beauty and strength. The Romans worshipped their athletes and their soldiers; children born defective were left on mountainsides to die. The first readers of this letter were suffering persecution and death. They were being mocked for compassionate values and derided for gentle character.

And so the author says, "Look into your own tradition to find your heroes—don't imitate the Roman values. Don't give in to popular definitions of worth. Don't admire someone who crucifies innocent people for political gain. The heroes in your own tradition," he writes, "gave up their own ambitions to administer justice."

I must tell you this morning that the HIV/AIDS community in America has gasped for the air of such justice. It has been scarred by discrimination and beatings, scars burned deeper by the message that those with HIV deserve the illness they suffer. Some have been tortured. Most have been jeered. They have been persecuted. They have been mistreated. It was so in ancient Rome; it is still so in modern America.

The only question is: What will those of us who have been surprised by grace in our own lives do for those most in need of grace today?

Perhaps you heard what the author said of those he calls heroes: Their weakness was turned to strength, but the world itself was not worthy of them.

Would you like to see where people turn their weakness to strength today? Come to a hospice for children with AIDS. Watch heroic staff and volunteers tease dying children and make them laugh. Walk with them to the lounge where, once through the door, the staff break down in tears and the volunteers hug themselves in grief. Are you amazed? Then look again. Because ten minutes later they go back out to the children, smiling, and they do it all over again. They collapse at night with the prayer, "My God, my God, why . . .?" And they come again the next day, and the next, to be a shepherd to the children and keep them from want. These are the ones of whom the world is not worthy.

Come with me to walk the streets of New York with a caregiver who, after a dozen years of life with this epidemic, has run low on patience with political arguments about condoms and needles. Two thousand times one man has posted funeral announcements on the bulletin board of his program. Two thousand times he has seen his work end at the grave. Two thousand times he has begged God for grace, and has somehow been surprised by it again. Here is a man of whom the world is not worthy.

Or come with me to my home. Stand with me in a corner of an early-morning kitchen while three-year-old Zachary plows into his cereal, spilling it all over his full-faced grin and his baseball pajamas. You who have tasted grace, whisper in my ear the word I should say to explain my future to Zachary. Give me a touch of your peculiar grace when my five-year-old, Max, says his friend's parent won't let him play with his friend's teddy bear. Share grace with me, and with our family, before anger consumes us and grief washes away whatever is left. Come be a hero in my life, one of whom the world is not worthy.

In a world that defines worth and value by our youth or our wealth or our power; in a world where we create quarterback heroes and beauty queen dreams—in this world where the standards have all been turned upside-down—we need to be surprised by grace in the shape of heroes, of whom the world is not worthy.

So here I am, a most ordinary person with what is rapidly becoming a most ordinary virus. Here I am, a representative of a community which has been lacerated by grief at every level. And here you are, a community of people who've been showered by a most extraordinary grace. Here we are together, at the intersection of grief and grace. Does it surprise you at all that I would ask of you, perhaps beg of you, to let that grace turn your weakness into strength? What's needed are congregations of heroes.

If you've tasted grace, it's easy. The AIDS community struggles yet with injustice and violence; join the struggle. To save our children we must fight ignorance and shame; join the fight. If you fear that association with the HIV/AIDS family will make you socially unclean; join the family. Be one of whom the world is not worthy.

Should anyone ask you why, explain that you are merely continuing an ancient tradition. You are following "the author of our faith who, for the joy set before him, endured the cross, scorning its shame. . . ."

Go, become one of whom the world is not worthy. Grace will go with you. And joy will follow you home.

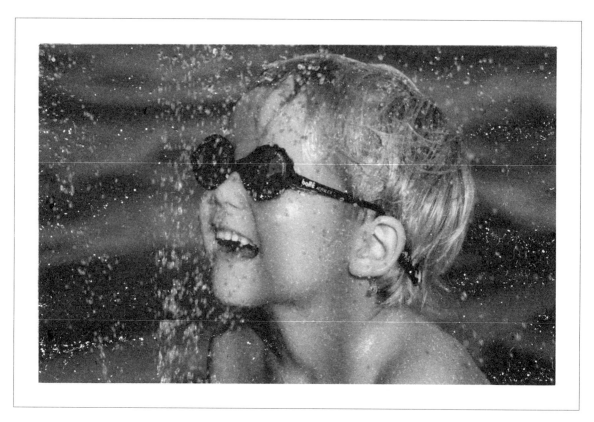

Thank God . . . Love, Willi

———o———

Betty Ford Center Alumni Dinner
Rancho Mirage, California
November 14, 1992

Betty Ford is more to me than a former First Lady or the name of a famous institution. She is not only a special friend; she's also my hero. She and President Ford are godparents for my first child—and, as it happens, were seated at the front table for this after-dinner speech.

In 1984 my mother completed treatment for alcoholism at the Betty Ford Center. As part of her treatment program, our family spent time at the Center. During that time, I decided that I'd complete the program for myself. It was a wonderful decision, leading not only to a clearer view of each day's miracles but also, through an art therapy ses-

sion, to the uncovering of whatever talents I may have as an artist.

No one is more at risk of AIDS than someone too drunk to make her own decisions or too high to control his own behaviors. But alcoholism treatment programs have often denied this risk, fearing (I suppose) that attention may shift from addiction to infection. Given the HIV virus "kill rate"— 100%—I've argued vigorously for AIDS testing and education as standard components of all such programs.

In my life, the nearest thing to apologizing to God is apologizing to President Ford . . . whom I always refer to as "*My* President."

My President made me the first woman advanceman in the history of the White House. I retaliated by subjecting My President to occasional indignities so he could learn the ancient truth: "No good deed goes unpunished." One of those incidents so mortified me that I've kept it secret for nearly two decades.

It was early in my White House career. I'd been up three nights straight trying to keep the peace between stubborn Secret Service agents, balky hotel managers, and even more stubborn advancemen. It's now late afternoon and hot and, during My President's fourth speech of the day, I may have dozed off for just a second or two. Suddenly, the speech is over, the agents are moving him toward me, we're late for the airport, people are shoving papers at me and My President leans down and whispers, "I'd like to use the men's room before we leave." So I lead him to the restroom, turn around, lean against a wall, and see the faces of the agents—mouths open—all aghast. Just as the door swings shut I hear a scream from inside the restroom: Clearly, a woman's voice. Clearly, twenty-seven years of habit had helped me send the President of the United States into an occupied woman's bathroom.

I've kept this quiet for almost twenty years, Mr. President, but Betty's got an honest program here; I need to respect the principles, tell the truth and make amends. So, Mr. President . . . I'm . . . I'm really sorry about that.

If I named every person in this room who deserves my thanks, the Academy Awards would seem short by comparison. One special person wasn't able to be here tonight, but I want you to know his irreplaceable contribution to my life. I met him, here, eight years ago. "My name is Willi," he said, "and I'm an alcoholic." So began my odyssey with Willi—spelled with an "i" at the end but no "e."

On the outside, you'd think—as I did at first—that Willi and I had nothing in common but alcohol: He, a black man and I, a white woman. He'd come up from poverty; I'd come out of privilege. He was cool and confident; I felt awkward and uncertain. He was tough and strong; I was frightened of myself, not yet strong enough to be vulnerable. When he saw something that was good, he'd explode, "Thank God!" When he stumbled over something hard in life, he'd mutter, "Ya' gotta' struggle."

The day he left, Willi sketched a pretty lady in the front of my book. I asked, "Who's that, Willi?"

"That's you," he said with a giggle. "Thank God!"

And in the front of my Big Book he wrote: "You are one of those people I know will be a friend. I can see the crazies in your eyes, and hear it in your laugh. Thank God! I hope your treatment here will keep you happy, healthy, and clean. Love, Willi."

Thank God for you, Willi; thank God for you so full of zest and energy and life, so willing to struggle, teaching me to struggle too.

Thank God for you, Willi; for you who cannot be here tonight because you lost the struggle with AIDS, and died.

It was here, somewhere between the comforting words of Betty Ford and the outstretched arms of Willi and you, that I learned who I am.

It was here that I gained the strength to be vulnerable so that, having faced the terror of my own weakness, I could grow strong. It was here that I learned to hand over control to God, so that He could become the Architect of my life—making of the wreckage I brought with me an amazing temple filled with songs of joy—sung, for the past five years, in the voices of my children.

A year ago last July I heard (as one hears a death sentence) that I was HIV-positive. The music stopped. I wandered in an empty canyon of time, shuttling from rage to despair to panic to self-pity. One day I opened my Big Book. "I hope your treatment here will keep you happy, healthy, and clean."

I began moving from anger to acceptance, hearing Willi say, "Ya' gotta' struggle."

I gave up feeling sorry for myself and learned to "Thank God!", Willi. I left the quiet corner where I was hiding to find a stage on which to tell the world, "I am not a victim; I am a messenger. Because in all things there is purpose." The lessons I learned here—from teachers as potent as Willi—eventually rescued me not once, but twice.

It's a rescue operation in which we might all become more expert, because the community of addiction—and, therefore, the community of recovery—is a community peculiarly and dangerously at risk. One-and-a-half or two million Americans are HIV-positive today. In ever-increasing numbers they travel the road to AIDS through every circle you and I inhabit: arts and entertainment, sports and business, government and finance, science and education. The virus has no political or economic, no ethnic or religious preferences; it enjoys being hosted by all. And none are more at risk than those too drunk to care. Given what we know from statistics about HIV, and what we know from experience about alcohol-saturated lives—anyone just now learning to say, "My name is Mary and I'm an alcoholic," is a person at risk for HIV.

If our goal is not merely sobriety, but health, we must come to grips with the epidemic which has become alcoholism's partner. Being sober is wonderful. But Willi's no longer sober, because Willi's no longer alive.

So I've come back tonight to apologize to My President, to say thanks to Willi—and to you—and to make a pledge on this, the tenth anniversary of this place of healing named for a woman I love: that I will not turn away from what most I detest in my own life, the virus, through which God is working His purpose for me. And I know I can keep this oath, because I see each of you keep your commitments one day at a time.

And, for years, I've seen it done by you, Betty. I remember the day you gritted your teeth at the surgeon's news. I heard you clear your throat and take the microphone. When women across this nation dared not breathe the words "breast cancer," when they hung their heads in fear and shame—I watched you climb the nation's rooftop and proclaim life over death. In speaking the words, you inspired a world to hope. In setting the model, you drained the terror and stigma. You did it not once, but twice. And you conquered more than cancer and more than addiction; you conquered the evils that were killing us.

If you look behind you, Betty, you will see a legion of us following in your footsteps: There's a pain-stricken young man just checking into the Center, proving that courage has not died. There's a contented grandfather, whose life was rescued late, showing what a life of quiet gratitude looks like. There's an unnamed mother whose children this morning rushed to hug her, sober, for the first time in a decade. There's an anonymous husband whose wife has dared at last to whisper, "I love you. I want you to come home." We are all here, Betty, following you, keeping our promises one day at a time.

And somewhere in the distance, if any of you would stand on your tiptoes and cup your ears, you could catch a glimpse of a most remarkable man. When the promises get hard to keep, you'll see him stretch out his arms to steady you and hear him say, "Ya' gotta' struggle . . . ."

And when you end the day sober—"happy, healthy and clean"—you may hear a quiet voice with a strangely familiar ring chuckling in the darkness: "Thank God. . . ."

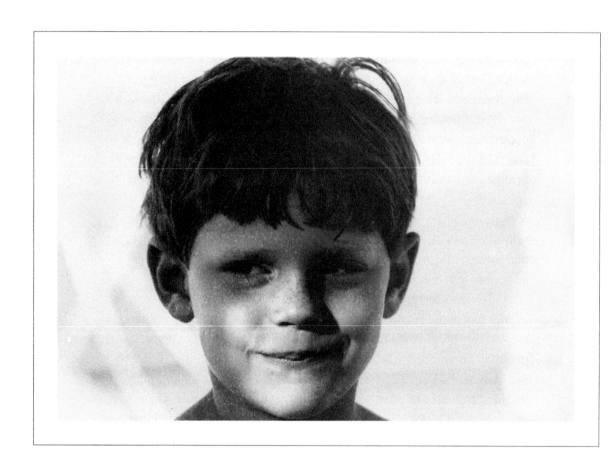

Remarks to the National Commission on AIDS

───────── O ─────────

Washington, D.C.
November 17, 1992

*During the final days of the 1992 presidential campaign the
rhetoric around AIDS grew especially shrill. The AIDS
community's leadership had moved into Clinton's camp. It came
as no surprise when Earvin Magic Johnson, earlier named by
President Bush to a post on the National Commission on AIDS,
sent a stinging letter of resignation and voiced his public support
for Governor Clinton.*

*In the wake of Magic's resignation, a few journalists called
to ask if I'd been contacted by the White House. They'd heard
rumors that I was being asked to serve. I'd heard nothing, and was
hopeful the post would remain vacant until after the election—
letting some of the political air out of the media balloon.*

*I was in Santa Fe visiting Sally Fisher in early October. We'd
gone for a sunrise walk in the clear desert air and returned to a*

message from my mother on Sally's answering machine: "So I've been watching you on CNN every half-hour—what else haven't you told me lately?" The President had casually mentioned, on national television, that he planned to name me.

The election was history by the time I was sworn in as Commissioner. I took the occasion to describe a vision of national leadership, a vision still not realized.

Veteran members and seasoned observers of the Commission know how limited is the power of this body. I'm aware of those limits myself, having spent most of my adult years covering, or being involved with, government organizations. I recognize that we are long on good intentions and short on authority. We have great power to proclaim and none to legislate. If we fail, we become just one more bureaucratic beast of burden braying in the Beltlined wilderness.

This Commission already has a record of outstanding service. If it were not so, you'd not have been so much debated during the recent election dialogue. I've always held the greatest respect for this body, not only for its work but also its character. Drs. June Osborn and David Rogers have been your colleagues while they became my friends and heroes. So I join you with a sense of humility at how much you've already achieved and how little I might add.

I bring with me a deep regard for public service and the personal convictions that should shape it. Rooted here is my belief that a Commission such as this has a potential greater than legislation, and a role more critical than budget-drafting.

We are the voice that must speak to the nation. We must speak thoughtfully, boldly, and consistently. We must keep the trust where there is still suspicion. And we must speak recognizing that we speak for others. Who else will represent the hundreds of thousands of grieving loved ones, if not we? True, we must speak *to* these fellow-

Americans; but we must also speak for them. We are named to be their voice. And if we are silenced; if we shade the truth for political or personal gain; if we lower our voice when we hear the distant thunder of a political storm—then we have failed not only at public policy but, worse, at public trust.

If you—if *we*—can speak convincingly to the soul of America, then we will be focusing on the issue at its deepest level. If we can be a compelling voice calling on the nation's conscience, it will be a visit that is long overdue. The calls to hatred and meanness have been heard too frequently, and too recently, for us to ignore. Dressed out in language of religion and morality, they have espoused a position worthy of neither.

And now is the time to join the issue, because signs are everywhere that the nation's conscience is restless on this issue. Judgmentalism, though not dead, has lost its easy appeal; it does not swagger across American communities as once it did. Compassion, though not yet triumphant, has gained at least a toehold in places where once it was a stranger.

Because speaking to the conscience can change the context in which my children may live without me, I can think of no mandate more urgent or valuable.

I've come intending to support aggressive research. I will continue to urge a complete and adequate government response, and full funding for it. I will be relentless in the search for a private-public partnership by which to make our efforts finally successful. And I am honored to do these things from a seat at the table you've already set with courage and distinction. But to press for better legislation without calling for greater dignity; to ask for more funds for HIV-positive citizens without challenging the immorality of the abuse they routinely suffer; to issue brave calls for government action without equally courageous calls to our fellow-citizens—

these would call into question our own understanding of the issues.

And so I join you, hoping my service will be worthy of you. It is my plan to listen much and speak little. But if there is a moment when the voice of one more HIV-positive person would make a difference, I would be happy if the voice were mine. I cannot extend or even save my life, but I can contribute it. And I am grateful to contribute it here, among you, in a pursuit you have already made honorable and with a voice that is already recognized for integrity.

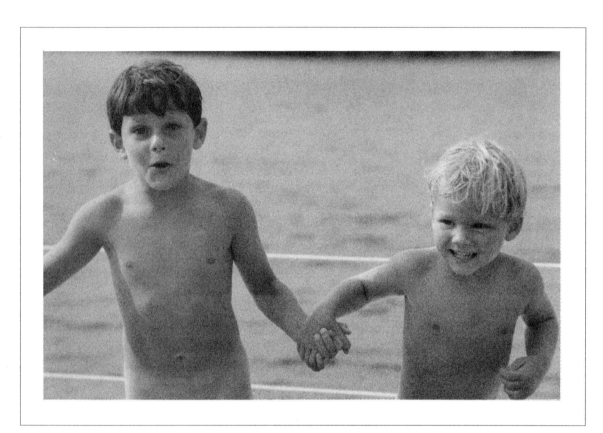

Make Me No Hero

———————————O———————————

Town & Country Award Dinner
New York City
December 2, 1992

*By the close of 1992 I was keenly aware of two problems:
People believed the myth about who gets AIDS, and I was
becoming a hero.*

*The myth says that only gay men and drug users get
AIDS. So, if I'm not gay and I don't use drugs, I'm not at risk.
This myth has made women, children and adolescents the
fastest growing HIV-positive populations. I needed to find
ways to say, "It isn't true," even if I could only make my
point by saying, "Look at me."*

*But the personal publicity which had at first let me
spread my message was, increasingly, becoming blurred by
an unrealistic caricature of me as a hero. I was no longer*

sure that inviting people to "look at me" was such a good idea.

When Town & Country *put me on its cover and made AIDS its December 1992 cover story, I was grateful. The magazine's readership is precisely the audience that most needs to hear the warning about risk and the call to community leadership. But, especially when the magazine honored me with its "Most Generous American Award," my fears of unwarranted hero-worship became clearer.*

The award dinner in New York was a wonderful event. My art was on display, my family and friends were there— Byron Nease took a night off from "Phantom of the Opera" in Toronto to sing for us in New York—and it was scheduled to be my last speech in 1992. It was, I thought, the right time to explain that I am not a hero.

Nineteen ninety-two has been a most extraordinary year for me and this evening is its capstone. I began the year coming to grips with being HIV-positive, plagued by the question: "Should I go public?" Good friends gave conflicting advice. We do not yet know who was right and who was wrong. Those of you who feared harm to our family have, thus far, thank God, been wrong: For the most part, we've done well as a family.

I may never know if going public was the right decision. But I made the decision for two reasons: Their names are Max and Zachary.

Like you, I do not know how many years I have before me. But I know how many children I have beside me.

Five-year-old Max will one day ask about his mother. And his brother, Zack, just two years younger, will pose all the same hard questions. Even if I could run from the press and hide from the public, I could never run or hide from them.

And so I went public knowing that, sooner or later, they would pass judgment on me. They would wonder if I had run from my own fears, or faced them; if I had avoided the hard questions, or accepted them; if I had merely praised good values, or had lived them; if I had struggled to improve their lives, or had abandoned them. It was not heroism that drew me into the public limelight in February; it was fear. I did not want to fail my children.

There was much I did not know when you published that first frontpage story in *The Detroit Free Press,* Frank Bruni*. I knew some people would wag their fingers and others would sneer behind closed drapes. But if I focused too much on the wagging fingers then, it was because I did not know there would be so many open arms; and if I dreaded too much the humiliation, it was because I did not yet understand that humility is a useful virtue. It takes away the fear that somehow you will be seen for what you are.

Some of the discoveries I made during 1992 were painful. I was certain, when I began, that people of good will would respond eagerly to an honest appeal. I was wrong. I had underestimated the political and economic forces involved in death and dying. I had overestimated the value we place on a single human life; we told the nation one-and-a-half or two million of us are HIV-positive, and they went on to the next story. And I'd grossly miscalculated the evil some would visit on this nation's gay communities, if they could.

I crisscrossed America during 1992 and discovered deep pools of prejudice and broad pockets of cruelty. The value of the discovery is that it has helped me position myself. I know something about myself now, which I'd never otherwise have known: I would rather reach for the

---

*Frank Bruni—*The Detroit Free Press* writer who authored the first story on my HIV-positive status (published February 13, 1992).

wasting hands of gay men and poor women who share this disease than be distanced from them by the label "innocent victim"—as if the means by which the virus first found us gave me some special purity, or cost them theirs.

Some of the year's discoveries about myself were hard. When I began, I thought I had completely come to grips with my HIV status. I'd moved from anger to acceptance. I'd given up focusing on dying from AIDS and taken on the challenge of living with HIV. But as the months wore on, I found that the process is not a straight line: We don't move from a temporary place of agony to a permanent state of commitment. Instead, we loop back; the process is a circle or, at best, a spiral. The demons who haunted my first terrorized nights still visit when I cannot sleep. The fear of losing my children hasn't disappeared; it finds me when I am tired and uncertain. The anger I thought I'd conquered flashes when least I expect it. And, just when I've urged others to replace judgment with compassion and prejudice with tenderness, I feel my own intolerance rising.

And some of the year's surprises were stunningly joyful. In wrestling with my own mortality, I discovered a new delight in each morning's sunrise. As my awareness of God's role in my life opened, I discovered that grief runs squarely into grace—and, in any contest between grief and grace, grace wins. In the tear-brimmed eyes of a young Utah woman, so collegiate and so grief stricken, whose father had died of AIDS, I discovered the healing that can flow from a long hug. In struggling to open my own heart and pour it out, I discovered someone who could read my soul and tell me the words. I must tell you that relationships are sweeter; my mother's late-night call is kinder; and to feel a loving hand slip into mine, this is ecstasy beyond description.

This was a year in which my heart learned to remember. If you could listen to my heart's memories from this year, you'd hear the rasping voice of a dying prostitute and the angry cries of an ACT-UP teenager. You'd hear *The New York Times*'s Jeffrey Schmalz challenging old stereotypes and June Osborn calling for new legislation. You'd hear the muffled sobs that seemed to rise from the AIDS Quilt itself as it was unfolded at the foot of the Washington Monument.

If you could listen to my heart, you'd come with me behind the scenes at Houston—not to the stage where I was much reported, but to the staircase behind the podium, where a reporter who'd asked such brittle questions in the morning stood sobbing, uncontrollably, barely able to say, "My brother just died of AIDS."

You'd come with me to North Carolina, to the little Methodist church where those of us who'd lost loved ones—parents and lovers, men and women, black and white—stood praying together, hugging together, weeping together as the choir sang "Amazing Grace."

If you could listen to my heart, you'd hear the sounds of playing children. You'd hear Max calling, "Mom—where are you, Mom?" and Zachary heading through the side door to explore the oversized ears on the neighbor's over-sized dog. You'd hear us saying "I love you" on the way to bed and "sleep with the angels" as the lights go out.

If you could listen to my heart, you would hear the song of a grateful mother and ordinary—very ordinary—woman.

When this year began, I feared that people would make of me a victim. I worried that, if I told my story in public, the public would treat me to pity. What I fear most now is not being translated into a victim, but being turned into a hero.

I am grateful for this gracious award and this wonderful evening. But if I had only one request to make this evening, it would be simple: Make me no hero.

You must remember that I did not volunteer for this fight: I was drafted, along with every other HIV-positive person in the world. I did not march bravely to the head of the line of duty; I was dragged into this arena, kicking and screaming. And many are the nights when I still scream, kick off the covers, and rush to my children's rooms for reasons I still don't understand.

If you need a hero, look to those who had no private purpose when first they stood in public and challenged their communities' patterns of prejudice and discrimination. Heap praise on those with moral courage who stubbornly refused to turn away from suffering and injustice. Save some award for the aging grandmother who, barely able to walk, still mounts the stairs to the local hospice and reads newspapers to blinded AIDS patients. Decorate with glory the father who cannot understand his 30-year-old son's story, but loves him enough to lift him onto the bed, wipe his fevered cheek, and bend low to say, "I love you, son."

And, here's the place I was surprised by grace: 1992 was a year in which I met thousands of such heroes, from New York to New Mexico, from the first phone call after my story was published to the last time I glanced around this room.

After such a year, and such an evening, it's no wonder that if you listened closely to my heart tonight, you'd hear it murmuring a song of thanks. And over the murmur you would hear, "I love you . . . sleep with the angels."

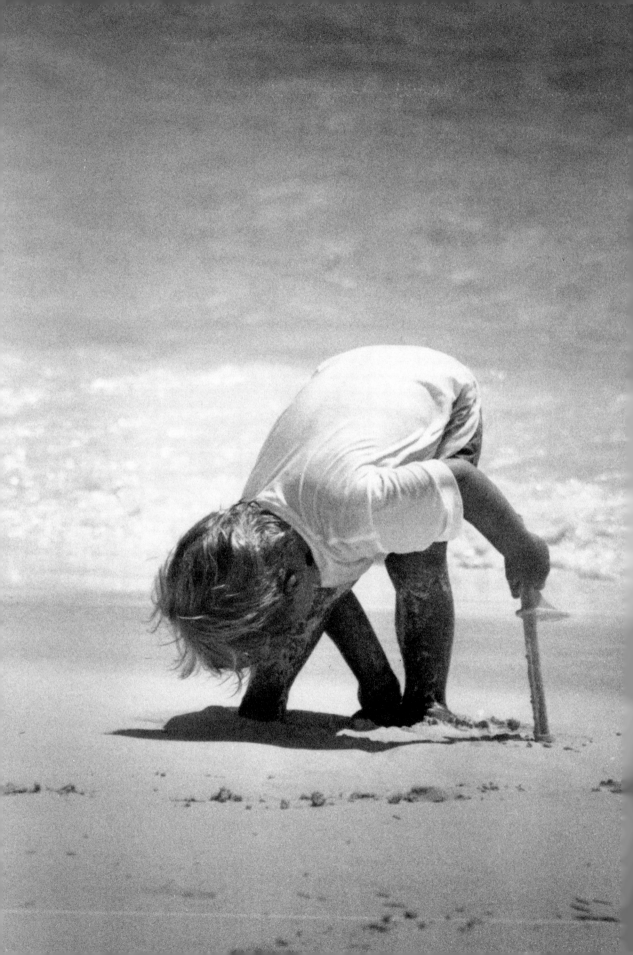

Reaching for the Hand of God

———————o———————

Women's Coalition of Memphis
Memphis
January 14, 1993

From the Town & Country *dinner until mid-January, I delivered no public speeches. It gave us time to look back on what had happened and lay plans for the months ahead. We decided to let the speeches run a little longer, where that was appropriate, and to pull no punches on the hard topics—from public policy to personal intimacy, including spirituality wherever possible.*

I was invited to Memphis by a women's civic coalition that hadn't worked together before. It included leaders from the African-American and Jewish communities as well as the local Junior League. When the audience was finally in place—in a huge, high school auditorium—I looked over a diverse community: men and women of all ages and races.

There were two electric moments in Memphis. The first came as everyone stood and held hands at the close of the speech; when I concluded, strangers who'd held each other's hands hugged and wept together. The second came when they surprised me with an award after I'd spoken. The award was a plate made by a local artist who came forward to present it. As he climbed the stairway to the stage, we all fell silent as the pain and weakness of his own AIDS became obvious. He gave me his gift of art. And then we—who, like the others, had been strangers—also embraced with tears.

Less than twelve months ago, in February 1992, I first disclosed publicly that I was HIV-positive. Tonight—January 14—could well be the one-year anniversary of my decision to "go public." After intense discussion with family and friends, and a good deal of soul-searching, the decision had finally been made not on grounds of psychology or politics, but on the basis of faith and family. I wanted my children to know that in all things in life there is a purpose; that if we are able to find the hand of God, and hold it, we can go anywhere; and that apart from God's hand, there is nothing else worth holding onto.

1991 had ended with echoes of a doctor's quiet voice telling me I was moving toward AIDS; this past year, 1992, ended in quiet reflection on how good God had been to me. This is my first public appearance in 1993. I hope you'll tolerate some reflections which may be a bit more personal than you expected. But I'd like to tell someone—and you all seem to be available—five lessons of acceptance I learned, some of them not for the first time, in recent months.

Lesson One: Life can be accepted as a precious gift.

When I was first told that I was HIV-positive, I couldn't imagine it. It wasn't possible. I'd never been at risk.

But reality settled in behind denial, and with it came a sinking depression that left me preoccupied with my own death. I imagined my parents, trying at their age to accept not only my death, but my death with AIDS. When I looked at my children, I could only see them as orphans. I spent more hours than I want to remember clinging to them, rocking them through long, dark nights. "Why me?" I kept asking. "Why me?"

Those of you who've hit rock-hard moments may know that question firsthand. We fear death. We fear being alone. We grope for comforting answers to discomforting questions. From the moment of conception and the hour of birth, our lives slope toward the grave. Some day, we will die. Even in the best of times—during the holidays, ending a hectic day, slumping at last toward bed—we can strangle our confidence and lose all hope of sleep by conjuring up the hard question: "What if I die tonight?"

In 1992, I discovered a harder question: "What if I don't die? What if I live? *Then* what?" What will I do in private with my children; what will I do and say publicly, here, with you?

We cannot save our own lives. I can't, and neither can you. Your life, like mine, is a gift. You may cling to it as tightly as you wish, as tightly as I tried to; it won't matter. You are neither the giver nor the keeper of your own life.

It's a humbling recognition to see that you and I are not, finally, in charge of our own lives.

But it's also a very freeing recognition, because it helps us set priorities. It helps us see that life is a great gift we have been given.

Lesson Two: We are enriched if we accept others as God's gift to us.

I'm not sure what seed of meanness was first planted in the human race. But its flower is evident. Because when we see others who are different than ourselves, we are prone to see them not as dissimilar in some regard, but as *less than*.

No social engine has ever been produced which so systematically, so brutally, and so long wore down a people as slavery. Stripped of history, down to the identities of our own parents; ripped apart through sale of children and mates; beaten bloody and pickled with salt if ever we raised our heads in dignity—we who are African Americans were not seen as different; we were seen as "less than." To be black was to be less than human.

No hand-hewn smokestacks have ever belched the stench of death with more ferocious hatred than those which rose over the treetops of Auschwitz. Parents and children were herded from cattle cars to the ovens. Names were replaced by tattoos; starvation and torture took the place of worship and hope. One-by-one they took us, until they took us by the millions. We who are Jewish were not seen as different; we were seen as "less than." To be Jewish was to be less than human.

Generations of women were told that they should hold their tongues and keep their place. And we were told what place had been reserved for our gender: We are followers, we were told, not leaders. Nurses, not doctors; teachers, not superintendents; secretaries, not presidents. We who are female were not seen as different; we were seen as "less than."

No community in America has been the subject of more brutal conversation or the object of more consistent abuse than those who are gay. For the same reason that tortured children take refuge from their abusers in some darkened closet, gay men and women have feared coming out. We who enjoy the majority have found in this minority a group to be hounded and harassed: We have used humor and economics and even Scripture as instruments not of grace but of torture. We who are gay are not seen as different; we are seen as "less than."

If we were to shape our souls according to American public opinion, then the elderly and the feeble have less value than the young and beautiful; the poor and homeless are drains on a society; and those with AIDS deserve their fate. We who are vulnerable are "less than."

If we do not see others as gifts of God; if we cannot value them for what they are, as brothers and sisters; then we will not grieve for their sorrow, struggle to relieve their pain, or mourn their passing. It accounts for the clear evidence and inescapable indictment on our own generation: that so long as HIV haunted the veins of gay men, and we were not gay, we did not care. Our compassion leapt within us only when the virus leapt all the fences and invaded the communities we thought were safe.

This is lesson two: We are ourselves enriched when we accept others as our brothers and sisters. That is, after all, who they are.

Lesson three: We need not be victims.

I've learned that no matter what others say or think of us, we need not make victims of ourselves. Indeed, I've learned in 1992 to detest the term "AIDS victim" which has sometimes been used to describe me.

Victims are weak and powerless. They are passive, having others do for and to them. They are no longer responsible, because responsibility has been taken from them.

But nothing has been taken from me by the virus; something has been added. I detest HIV. But I am not its victim. It has not weakened my humanity, and it will not. It has not stripped my power as a person, and it can not. I'm responsible for me and my children, and I'm competent to meet my responsibilities. Some people *want* to be victims. But most of those in the community of HIV/AIDS deplore the label and the misunderstanding which it represents.

A great teacher on this subject is the man who knocked on the back door of Jim's home some years ago. My friend, Jim, opened the door to an old man with glassy eyes, a chin bristled by days of unshaven growth, and clothes in sorry need of repair. He clutched a wicker basket with some dirty vegetables he wanted to sell. Jim bought a few out of pity, and quickly, to move the man along.

But it did no good. Day after day the man came back. Jim discovered that his name was Mr. Roth, that he lived in a shack down the road, and that his glassy eyes were a consequence not of alcohol but of cataracts. He wore mismatched shoes—two left shoes, one brown and one black. When brought to the kitchen table for coffee, Mr.

Roth would—without coaxing—pull a harmonica from his torn trousers and play mournful gospel melodies.

One bitter winter morning, Mr. Roth appeared with a few squash and some good news. "A wonderful thing happened this morning," he told Jim. "I came out my back door and found a bag full of shoes and clothes sitting there."

"That's wonderful," Jim smiled, having left them there late the night before.

"Yup," said Mr. Roth. "But the *really* good news is that just yesterday I met some folks who could really use them."

Some of us here have been whipped by racism; we can be its victim, or its survivor. Some of us have been slandered by antisemitism; we now choose to be its victims, or its survivors. We have suffered for our gender or our sexuality, for our age or our poverty; we have suffered because we carry a virus. Okay. We've suffered. Now what?

I pray that when my children see me, they will see not a whimpering victim of society's mistakes, but a hopeful, determined survivor. And I offer the same prayer for you.

The fourth lesson I learned in 1992 is this: We must accept ourselves if we are to accept others.

I'll tell you the truth: This was the hardest lesson of the past year, perhaps of my life.

When the news came in 1991 that I was HIV-positive, I'd just begun to reassemble the pieces of my life after a divorce. My children were doing well. My art was great (even selling!). My friends and family were wonderful sources of joy. Then came the news.

I ran. I retreated into my home and buried myself in a few trusted relationships, living in terror that others might discover the truth. I closed doors to people who called. I closed doors to friends who asked what they could do. I curled up so tightly that no one could get in.

The person I blocked out most was me. I tightened against the pain. I fought to think of something else. I hated the voice I heard from deep within myself. It told me that HIV and AIDS are dirty; therefore, I was now a dirty woman. I could no longer think of myself as feminine. I had become "less than . . ."—HIV had made me less than a woman, less than desirable, less than capable of loving and being loved. I was a modern-day leper who should not be touched. I, who had always struggled for approval—from being high school class president all four years to being the White House's most perfect advance person—*I* was now infected with something that proved how unworthy, how unapprovable, I *really* was.

What finally touched me most deeply, what changed me most profoundly, was a deep and growing spirituality that introduced me to grace. Slowly, I came to the conviction that if God truly loves by grace—a gift he gives, not something we earn—then I can trust that, even in *this*, there is some good purpose. And I can accept myself as part of his will.

It's when I began to accept grace, that I began to accept myself, as I am—including HIV-positive—and that I began also to accept others back into my life again. Painfully, I discovered that we can accept others only when we can accept ourselves.

Which leads me to my final lesson, and it is this: We will live or we will die by what we love.

When the poet Wordsworth came to the end of his epic work, "The Prelude," he closed with this memorable text:

> What we have loved,
> Others will love,
> And we will teach them how.

If your children are like mine, they are great imitators. What you and I love, they will love; and we will teach them how.

Because I love my children, and want them to love me, this is a terrifying truth. What happens if I should need to leave them, and they are raised in a culture that teaches disrespect for those with HIV? What will they love, and who, if their models all say that AIDS is a disease which is deserved—that those who suffered and died of this virus were "less than . . ."?

I am not a historian, but I have visited slavery and felt the heat of Hitler's ovens. I've heard gay men and HIV-positive women confess their status with terror. Surely those of us who have descended from slavery understand the awfulness of being told that we are less than human. Those of us whose parents were tattooed by Hitler's troops, whose mothers were told they were not worthy, who've felt the sting of prejudice and oppression—surely, all of *us* can see the need for change; surely, we will stand with those who are oppressed . . .won't we?

My greatest fear is that the society in which my children grow will teach them, despite whatever relationship I develop with them, that their mother—because of AIDS—is unworthy. It would not be done intentionally, I suppose; but unintentional prejudice is just as deadly as that which wears white hoods and burns wooden crosses.

But I am not the only parent with fears related to AIDS. Perhaps you are, yourself, in that camp. I offer two simple pieces of advice: first, get factual information so that you are educated about the realities of HIV and AIDS. If you don't know where to get the information, ask, tonight; experts from the Memphis area are here and available to you.

Second—now take a deep breath—talk to your children. Ask them about HIV; tell them you worry about AIDS. Explain that you love them, and want them to stay alive. And don't worry about "not saying it right." In the most important moments of our lives, we often fumble our lines. It doesn't matter. What kind of love would we have for our children if, in the face of history's most deadly epidemic, we withheld the information that could save our children's lives? If you want to make notes for a conversation with your child, I can give you exactly the right opening words: "I love you . . . ."

As adults, as mates, if you have ever been at risk in any way, get tested. You do not need to be gay; you do not need to inject drugs; and you do not need to be promiscuous in order to be at risk. Believe me, I know about this. All you need to do—just once—is have a partner who—just once—took a chance with a risky partner or a risky behavior. The chains of relationships, in which every link can be infected, grow longer each day. If you think you may be at risk, for your own good and that of everyone you love, I urge you: Get tested. It's confidential. And it can be done for free.

It's my belief that our lives together, and our time tonight, is really not all about HIV or AIDS. At core, it is about love and grace. Because, in the end, we will not find ourselves reaching for another insight or another dollar, or even another cure. We will be reaching for the hand of God, wanting to be steadied as we pass from one life to another, wanting not to be left alone.

The nearest thing to the hand of God in this life is the hand of someone who loves you. It is the new mother's hand brushing gently along the back of her nursing newborn. It's the father's hand that lifts a tiny child high enough above the crowd to see the passing parade. It's the first time you held hands with someone who thought you were handsome, or pretty, who hoped for a good night kiss. It's the hand of a grandmother soothing her husband's fevered brow. It's your hands; reaching toward my children, when I can no longer lift my own hands to serve them.

Reach for the hand of God, and you will find joy. Until then, reach for one another, where you may also find grace and peace.

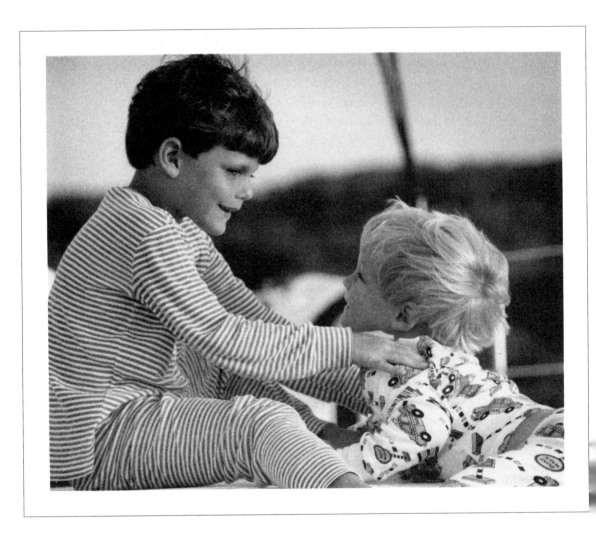

In the Valley of the Shadow

———————— O ————————

National Institute for Community Health Education
Hamden, Connecticut
March 3, 1993

While visiting New York for the Town & Country *dinner in early December, I'd joined mutual friends for a leisurely lunch with Arthur Ashe. We had lots to discuss and the time flew by quickly, closing with the usual promises to stay in touch and be well. Two months later, he was dead.*

Arthur had agreed to give a luncheon speech to several hundred healthcare professionals. I was asked (and agreed) to take his place. And I chose to hold back nothing—from anger to prayer—when I decided to talk about life in the valley of the shadow of death.

I am deeply grieved to be today's speaker. This was an appointment made by Arthur Ashe, not Mary Fisher, and I wish—more than you can imagine—that he had kept the appointment. He relished this sort of occasion because he loved to meet, and to challenge, those who are—as he was—bright and committed and concerned. His was a gentle voice of great wisdom, and I regret beyond words that you cannot hear that voice today.

The day of Arthur's funeral I told Jeanne, his wife, that so long as I could speak, Arthur's voice would be heard. But in the days that followed, I began to doubt the truth of my own attempt at comfort.

Atlanta Mayor Andrew Young said that he had called Arthur's home telephone number the day Arthur died, hoping to find Jeanne there. Instead, he got the answering machine with Arthur's voice saying, "I'm away for a minute; leave a message and I'll get right back to you."

In the hours and days, and especially in the nights following Arthur's death, it occurred to me that Arthur wasn't going to be right back. In fact, he is gone. In fact he is terribly, irrevocably dead. The reality of his death is especially chilling for those who were uniquely bonded to Arthur by HIV, those thousands of us who knew him a little and loved him a lot.

That incredible November day two years ago, when Magic Johnson gave his smiling, full-of-life-and-hope news conference, a shiver of joy ran through the AIDS community across this country. We were united not only with him, but with each other, in a moment of hope that lifted spirits for days to come. Again at the close of last year, when *Sports Illustrated* lifted Arthur to the top of the world, a bond of courage flowed over the AIDS community that was so strong you could feel it.

Then Arthur died. One would expect that the community which had been bonded by his courage would be united again in that moment. But it did not happen. The shiver of joy was replaced, instead, with a shudder of fear when we saw the stark, cold reality of his passing. In his death, we all saw our own dying. We saw the end of the road that we are traveling. We saw that all his fame and decency, all his grace and glory, could not save him. Holding Jeanne's hand may have comforted him, but it did not rescue him; and his daughter, Camera, will not be warmed by hugging trophies in the night. Arthur was larger than life, but not larger than death. And in the wake of his dying I have spent nearly a month wandering in what the ancient psalmist described as the "valley of the shadow of death," feeling, in ways I've never felt before, alone.

I did not come to depress you today. But neither did I come to spare you. I want you, who have devoted yourselves to the care and healing of others, to know the importance of your devotion. When you leave today, I hope you take with you a renewed sense of the importance not only of what you do but also, more urgently, the importance of who you are.

Let me take you back a few days before Arthur died. On Wednesday, February 3rd, we began hearing early reports of a study by the National Research Council of the National Academy of Sciences. The study was released the next day under the title "The Social Impact of AIDS in the United States."

When the study was released, the chair of the Council summarized the findings in these words, and I quote: "AIDS has devastated the personal lives and social communities it has touched, but the epidemic has had little affect on American society as a whole or its way of doing business."

Under a deluge of scrutiny and criticism, the report's authors subsequently explained that they had not intended to say that AIDS was unimportant; they had only meant to say that it was largely invisible. They had meant only to point out that most people who are HIV-positive are from "socially marginalized" groups.

The truth is: AIDS has left America's gay communities and the nation's hemophiliac community in ruins. The community of arts and letters has been impoverished by the loss of playwrights and photographers, poets and dancers and musicians. We have lost legislators and legal experts, physicians and researchers, mothers and fathers and tiny children of unknown potential. And so far, we have only lost about 10% of those who have contracted HIV in America; the other 90% of us who are HIV-positive are here, living out our lives—socially marginalized or not. The raging epidemic of infections has taken barely a tenth of the toll it would wreak *if there were a perfect preventative today.*

There is currently no cure, and no preventative. So we move ahead with darkened stages in the wake of dead playwrights, naked walls where vibrant photography might have been. Our hours are silent, where once they were stirred by the poet's voice and the performer's song, both now stilled. We will never again see the dancer leap who, not long ago, leapt so high—and froze there, in the air, as if by magic—and floated back to us from his magic heights. Are these the ones who are "socially marginalized"? Is it they who are invisible?

Dr. David Rogers, Cornell Medical Center's longtime leader, a mentor for all of us on the National Commission, and America's foremost spokesman on AIDS, responded to the report with a personal letter to the chairman. He sent me a copy and I hope he doesn't mind this public use of his private thoughts. This is part of what Dr. Rogers—perhaps the mildest man I know—said to the report's author:

"[Y]ou told every major corporation and every conservative American institution exactly what they wanted to hear. 'HIV/AIDS will disappear. . .because those who continue to be affected by it are socially invisible, beyond the sight and attention of the majority population.' Their reaction is, 'Hot dog!' . . .Now all of us on the front lines are suddenly faced with damage control and trying to deal with what I find is the prevailing attitude: 'Thank God it's them, not us; now we can go back to business as usual and forget about those folks.' "

A month later, I am less discouraged than angry. I'm angry because David Rogers proved to be right. Radio talk show hosts had a field day with the report, using it as clear evidence that there is no epidemic worthy of the nation's attention and priorities. That troubles me.

Some politicians used the report to justify their opposition to increased support for AIDS research and to maintain their prejudices, so well nurtured over the past dozen years. That troubles me.

Advertisers who pay for media stories have once again been given a reason not to sponsor programs dealing with HIV and AIDS, thus maintaining the silence that has helped to kill us. That troubles me.

But I am troubled even more by the quiet teenager who read the story somewhere in mid-America and decided that she was no longer at risk with the boyfriend she admires more than she knows. I was stung by a pain that has converted to anger, that after thousands of hours of work and millions of dollars of effort to bring awareness and sensitivity, one insensitive report can put at risk young people across the country.

I cannot give enough speeches to undo that damage. And the authors' innocent intent, which I accept, does not undo it either.

The report went public on Thursday. A journalist from one of America's most prominent newspapers interviewed me that day. At one point in the interview, I expressed irritation at the consequences of the report—a softer and less reasoned version of what you just heard from me here. She was quick to say, "Mary, this isn't a report about you. You're the exception. This is a report about most people with HIV." Nothing has troubled me more than this.

Do you know how it feels to be exempt from the group which offers you a primary part of your identity?

"You're a Native American? Well, Mary, you're not like the others; you're a good Indian."

How does it feel to be separated from your family, only to have your family maligned?

"You're a Jewish woman? Well, Mary, you're not like those kikes; you're a good Jew."

Do you hear the sound of that? Can you feel me being lifted away from those I love so that I'm not hit when the firing starts?

"You're an African-American? Well, Mary, you're not like the others; you're a good nigger."

Does the language offend you? Does it make *you* angry? It should. But it is not just the language which should offend; even more, it is the ugliness of discrimination, the brutality of judgments. If we are human, such evil should awaken in us a terror and commitment that the AIDS movement has not yet seen in this nation.

If those of us who are HIV-positive could draw no other lesson from Arthur Ashe's death, then we should draw this one: No one in the HIV/AIDS community is exempt. No one. No matter who you are, what you have, or how nicely folk describe you—if you are HIV-positive, you are *not* exempt. We are, all of us, part of a one- or two-million-person pilgrimage, kicking up dust as we move clumsily but certainly toward an unhappy end. Magic Johnson is not exempt. Mary Fisher is not exempt. No one is exempt. We are, all of us, part of the group branded "invisible," "socially marginal," lacking impact—which is to say, in straightforward language, that we are part of a group which has not yet mattered to America.

This past holiday season a kindergarten child spent nearly a week of time making his mother an ornament. With every ounce of dexterity five-year-old fingers could muster, he'd made of toothpicks and tiny crystal figurines a delicate masterpiece which would grace the family's mantel. The last day of school before vacation, parents were invited in to pick up their children—and to get their ornaments. When he saw his mom and dad coming, he couldn't restrain himself. He went dashing through the crowd of children and, just short of his parents, he tripped and fell and the ornament was shattered in a thousand hapless pieces.

His father, loving him deeply and sensing the enormous hurt, bent over and whispered, "It doesn't matter, it doesn't matter. Mommy knows you love her." But his mother, in a moment of wiser grace, picked him up and cried with him, saying, "I know, I know, it matters. It matters very much."

I want to say something to you that I have never, never, *never* said in public before. I've hardly been able to say it in private. But I want you to hear me say it, and I want you to remember that I said it when you go home: I matter.

I do not matter because my name is Mary Fisher and I've talked on some stages. I matter because my children call me Mom, because my artwork is a gift, because a friend said "I love you" on the telephone this morning. I matter because I am still alive, and I am still human. It's the same reason my children's father, who may be less well known, matters. He is human. He matters.

And so do you. If in your work you are able to nurture them for an hour, it matters very much. If in your strength you can give them hope; if in your wisdom you can give them good judgment; if in your healing and your hugs you can give them self-acceptance and encouragement—all of this matters. It matters, very much.

I know how tired you must become of working with us, sometimes. We all grow tired of living in the valley of the shadow of death. Caregivers grow weary of fighting their own emotions and healers are weakened by too many struggles, too many crises, too many losses along the way. We—you—want to retreat, go home, take up a cause or career with great financial reward. You grow weary of helping people die, eventually, and you want to go away. I understand. There have been too many hours, especially in the past month, when I wanted to climb out of the valley myself and it no longer seemed to matter whether I climbed out by living or by dying.

I will make a pact with you this morning. If you will not give in to the temptation to look away from those who suffer, I will not give in to the temptation to merely be angry. Then, neither of us will need to go away. Together, we can affirm that we matter.

I have three special appeals today. They are brief. And they're personal. But I think they're important.

First, I wish that in your work you would pay special attention to the women who are HIV-positive or at risk of being HIV-positive. I care no less about men than women, but women have faced some special struggles with this disease.

Typically, they struggle because their communities may not have a natural support group able to carry them over the most difficult spots. When the disease was first identified, gay communities in which it had such devastating consequences rallied with strong agencies of care and support. Now, as the epidemic moves into increasingly young, hetero-sexual, and female populations, such community structures are often lacking. Be sensitive in such communities to women's need for support. Without it, many will fear even to be tested—even when they know they have been at risk. And those already living with knowledge that they are HIV-positive often survive by telling no one. They fear that disclosure will cost them their employment, their insurance, perhaps even their children.

Women have a fear which is almost never discussed: an extraordi-nary dread of lonesomeness. It is the fear that we will be left alone and isolated, never again hugged or loved, never again given esteem or value, let alone a sense of being virtuous. It is the fear that AIDS is so "dirty" a disease that all who have it are dirty too. Were it not so private a topic, I could speak of this lonesomeness with an eloquence born of personal agony. The fear that we have become unlovable is a potent fear, and when the fear itself is reinforced, we are immobilized.

You need to tell HIV-positive women that they are no less women simply for having this virus. If they were worthy as mothers before, they are worthy now. If they were loving sisters and caring friends before, they are so now. If they were trusted lovers and wives before, they can be trusted no less today. HIV will do damage enough. We must not let it destroy women early by taking away their own sense of themselves as beautiful, worthy and desirable.

Second, I appeal to you to raise your voice on behalf of those who are silent. In the wake of the last presidential elections, an interesting thing has happened: A hush has fallen over the national AIDS community.

I think I understand this silence. I suspect it is borne of a misunderstanding which was prevalent during the election itself. Then, many in the AIDS community believed that the problem was President Bush; if only he could be changed, the nation would be changed. If Bush was the problem, Clinton is the solution. It was a bad analysis last fall and it's bad logic this spring.

I pray for the President's success in every regard, but he cannot change the nation's priorities on his own. It's the Senate that just voted to sustain immigration sanctions against HIV-positive people. It's senators and legislators in state as well as federal offices who need to be sensitized—who tell me, when I speak to them, that they'd like to help but, "well, nobody in my district is really affected by this problem." We need to remember that Washington tends to follow the nation in setting priorities; it does not lead them. A change in the White House is not enough. What's needed is a change in all the other houses in America— in your home and mine, and in all the homes of our neighbors.

And so I appeal to you to stand up and speak out on behalf of the AIDS community. If you fear being branded as one who loves gays and identifies with the "socially marginalized," you would be wiser to confront your fear than to give in to it. Because the day will come when America will fully understand how little this virus cares whether you are gay or straight, male or female, rich or poor. As someone said last August in Houston, "This virus asks only one thing of you: 'Are you human?' And that is the right question: 'Are you human?' "

Finally, I want to appeal to you to have faith. And I do not mean this either as some kind of weak piety or a call for you to believe what I believe. But it is, nonetheless, an appeal for you to have faith. And I appeal for this because, in the valley of the shadow of death, I do not know what else will sustain us.

At Arthur's hometown funeral in Richmond, Virginia, we all stood and read from Psalm 103. Not only was this his favorite psalm. It also contains a description of the Arthur whose patience on the tennis court and in life was legendary: "The Lord is merciful and gracious," wrote the psalmist, "slow to anger and plenteous in mercy." Slow to anger. That was always Arthur.

My own favorite psalm, one I learned as a child, is the Twenty-Third.

The Lord is my Shepherd, I shall not want;
He maketh me to lie down in green pastures.
He leadeth me beside the still waters; he restoreth my soul.
Yea, though I walk through the valley of the shadow of death,
I will fear no evil; for thou art with me . . . .

I have long believed, and consistently said, that in all things there is divine purpose. I do not pretend to understand God's ways, but I believe that even my being HIV-positive is within the divine plan. And I draw comfort from that.

But I draw more comfort from the ancient poet's promise that I am not alone in the valley of the shadow of death. Trained to think of God as some distant and powerful king, I am encouraged to think of Him also as a fellow-traveler. I have come to think of God as walking among us—

walking with, say, a million or two million pilgrims kicking up dust as we move clumsily but certainly along.

And when the whole company of pilgrims stops because someone at the lead has fallen; when a whisper comes down through the crowd that "Arthur has died"; when, at that moment, we look to the edge of the crowd and see God, bent over, weeping, then we have come to the moment of faith. It is in the valley of the shadow of death that we learn to cry not only to God, but also with him.

Arthur is gone. I cannot bring him back, nor can you. But if I, if we, look for meaning in his death, we are probably looking in the wrong direction. It's not in death that we learn the great lessons, it's in life.

When we learn the lessons by faith, we can take courage. We learn to walk the hard road to glory together, to struggle together, to weep together. With faith we will have less fear of touching the untouchable, less reluctance to reach out in comfort to those whose grief is still beyond comfort. It's a critical lesson for each of us to learn. Else it is not only the HIV-positive woman who will be terribly, terribly alone; it will be all of us.

Ultimately, this is our calling, yours as well as mine. We must find enough faith to go back to it, me, after this speech and, you, after this conference. We need to take up where we left off, channeling the emotions that will otherwise destroy us and wither our commitments. We need to look deeply into life, finding meaning in the embrace of our children and the knowledge that they, and we, matter. The pilgrim crowd needs to get moving again, enlarged, I hope, by some of you.

Earlier this year playwright Paul Rudnick was explaining in *The New York Times* (January 23, 1993) why gay writers have written comedies about AIDS: "Only money, rage and science can conquer AIDS," he said, "but only laughter can make the nightmare bearable."

If we can find faith to sustain us, and each other to hold us, we may yet—you and I—hear laughter over the tears. Until we all hear the laughter, I wish you God's grace.

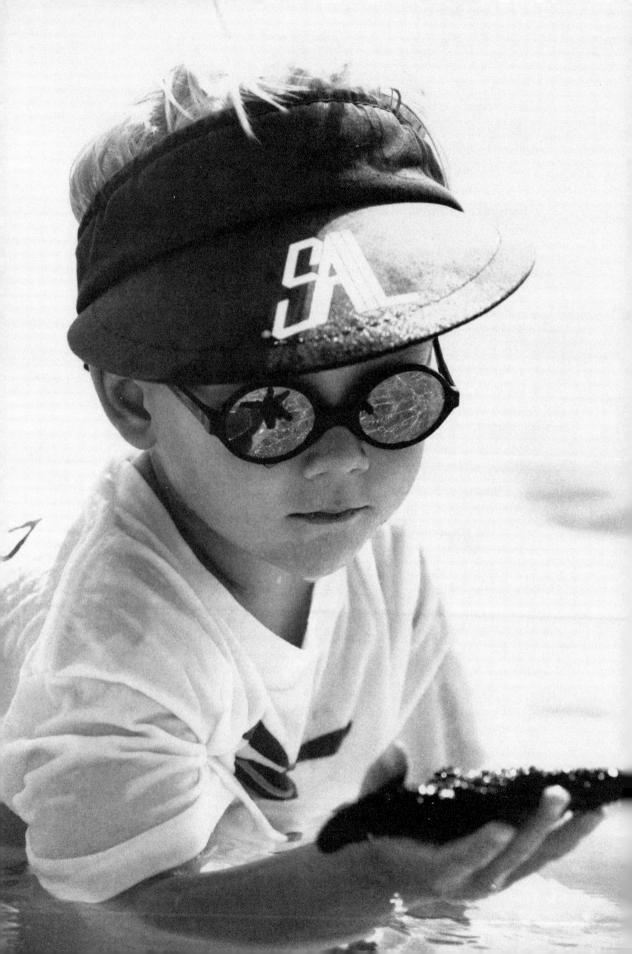

Intimate Conversations

———————O———————

Salem State College
Salem, Massachusetts
April 1, 1993

Salem State College has for some years hosted a distinguished community lecture series. Geoff Mason, a dear friend who lives near Salem, called me the day they took Arthur Ashe's name off the lecture series marquee and replaced it with mine.

I remember the evening of this speech vividly, because it was the only time that Brian—Brian Campbell, the man I'd loved and married and with whom I'd twice become a parent—heard me speak. He was living in Boston and was already sick, but when I accepted this date he said he wanted to come and sit with the children. In some sense, this was a speech I gave to Brian—an intimate, and probably overdue, conversation with the man whose AIDS I shared.

Brian came as promised. As the evening wore on, first Zack and then Max grew restless. Brian eventually stood up and carried them to the back of the auditorium. There they fidgeted in his arms until, nearing the end, I told the audience that when I tuck them into bed I tell them to "sleep with the angels." With that, Zack put his head on one of Brian's shoulders and Max rested on the other. Both went to sleep, with Brian slowly rocking them.

A thousand times or more that image has come back to me, especially a few months later at Brian's graveside.

A few people have come here this evening just for me: family members who knew me as a child, friends who've filled great portions of my life, people I've known and loved and sometimes feared I'd lost. This group is small in size but large in impact. Because they have known me offstage, intimately, what might otherwise be merely public address becomes personal conversation. We knew one another in other days, in other moments, before we knew the word "AIDS." And because you've come, we should talk. In fact, I want to say publicly what I've had a hard time saying privately, and to let others in on our conversation.

Some people have come tonight not because of me, but because of the virus I bear, although they do not bear it themselves. You are members not of the *in*fected community, but of the *af*fected. You are nurses who administer the tests and deliver the awful news, social workers who know the homes and hospices of the AIDS community, doctors whose knowledge has not yet been enough to stop this little killer. You are the sisters and the brothers, the parents and the lovers who've been left behind, or who dread the hour you will be. You bring laughter on good days, hugs on bad days, and hope when ours begins to falter. You are acquainted with a peculiar grief that begins long before the graveside. You've stood beside the bedside of someone you loved passionately, only to discover you had no words either to hold them or, harder still, to let them go. I'm glad you're here, and I hope you'll not mind letting others overhear my conversation with you.

Some people have come out of curiosity; you are welcome. Some came feeling responsible; I'm glad you're here. Some came feeling fear; you don't need to be afraid. But you do need to hear some of what is said here. In this group are the members of our community, the people with whom we share responsibility for life around us.

And some have come tonight because, like me, they are HIV-positive. They are here because, when there is no cure, you seek comfort in your illness; when there is no healing, you search for hope. Your presence is an act of solidarity, and I thank you. Those who've told others of their status can enjoy the support of others about them. If you've not yet told the truth in public, perhaps you'll find new hope and courage this evening. We must speak candidly to each other, those of us who are pilgrims on the road to AIDS. And we must not worry about those who listen in.

So here I am, a five-foot-one, blonde Republican. And there you are, an audience of wonderful diversity, four groups of listeners trapped in one auditorium: pilgrims who walk with me, fellow travelers who care for us, neighbors who share our community, and a little band of relatives and friends. I have no long speech, just four intimate conversations to share—and you may listen in when I'm speaking to the others.

If these were four letters, I would aim the first to those who are HIV-positive, and I would write to you as "My Fellow Pilgrims." You are part of a pilgrim band which numbers more than twelve million globally and one-and-a-half million or so in America.

You are the ones I've come to Salem to embrace, each of you. The reason I would embrace you is that life with HIV is often a life laced with lonesomeness. In an age of increased mobility, electronic communication, and breakdown of social convention, lonesomeness has become a common feature of modern life. But it is uniquely common among those who carry this virus. The root cause is stigma, the same sense of dread which has kept some here this evening from sharing the intimate truth about their HIV status.

For HIV-positive men, the stigma has sometimes attached to substance abuse which put you at risk. Often, it has attached to being gay. Some of you knew the meaning of "bashing" not only in a physical sense, but also in a familial sense. From your earliest memories to your latest, you lived a secret life. When you sought a sense of comfort, you discovered what discrimination was in store for you. Then came HIV. Like the Jews in Germany a half-century ago, you drew every breath waiting for discovery; but in your case it was double jeopardy, since either being gay or being HIV-positive might be enough to lose your job, your home, your independence, your sense of worth. And so you withdrew into a lonesomeness that pierces your soul and drains your joy.

For those of us who are women, the stigma has often been attached to a sense of being "damaged goods." We have uncovered a modern parallel to the old, ugly and false stereotype of alcoholics: "funny drunks" if they're men and "dirty whores" if they're women.

It is no doubt true that HIV and AIDS have drawn a shower of stigma and discrimination in most communities. Such patterns must be challenged and stopped. But you and I who are HIV-positive must be careful not to become victims. What we need to challenge mean judgments and vicious discrimination is power, not pity.

If for your HIV-status you are judged an unworthy parent, look to the eyes of your children to know your worth. If for your

HIV-status you are judged evil or wicked, let God be the judge and live life by his grace. If for your HIV-status you judge yourself inferior, a failure, a person not deserving of affection—you are injuring yourself without cause. I have a suggestion for you: Stop.

Perhaps the lesson we most need to learn is that of forgiveness. We have family members who do not understand that we did not seek this disease; that we were drafted to be pilgrims on this road, we did not enlist; that we did not set out to embarrass them or injure ourselves. If we wish to move on, we cannot wait to convert them all; we will need to forgive them.

We can spend our life in anger at a tainted needle, or an unsafe American blood supply, or an undetected virus in someone we loved. Or we can set aside the anger in favor of forgiveness, and move on.

We can live our lives regretting the moment we were not careful; we can consume our children with our own guilt at leaving them; we can hate ourselves until there's nothing left worth saving. Or we can learn to forgive ourselves as well as others.

This is neither pop psychology nor cheap grace; it is merely living out the ancient hope that we will one day learn how to pray, "Forgive us our debts, as we forgive our debtors."

Dear Pilgrim, if you need to hear a word of forgiveness, hear it now. The road is hard enough and we will grow weak too soon. It isn't possible to take this journey weighed down. We must forgive even ourselves, reach out to take another's hand, and move on. Else we will be not a company of pilgrims but a crowd of pitiful victims. God forbid. And God give us strength.

I do not want to be maudlin; HIV is unpleasant enough, and AIDS wrings out our lives too soon. But neither do I want to be romantic about those who serve us. And here, in public, in a community that prides itself on service to others, I want to say to the caregivers present: You are God's angels in our midst.

If you would like to see the angels at work, you merely need to look around you. Look at the agony on the face of the woman whose task, day in and day out, is to convince HIV-positive mothers to sign over their children. Who but an angel would infuse her profession with love for those she serves, knowing her love will end in grief? Who but a saint would commit his career to clients or patients whose best future is uncertain? It is backbreaking labor to turn bodies in the night, even when they have withered. It is heartbreaking work to turn pages of one's address book to see name after name after name, all scratched out, all gone.

It is no wonder that hardly an AIDS conference can be held in America today without sessions on "professional burnout." It's understandable. And I have no easy solution for those of you who grow weary of caring for those of us who grow weary of needing care.

But if you have sometimes wondered if it is all worthwhile; if you have thought to yourself that it makes no difference whether you serve one more person with AIDS; if in the night, when you lie awake, it all seems overwhelming—I have a story for you first told in Loren Eiseley's "The Star Thrower." A young man was picking up objects off the beach and tossing them out into the sea. A second man approached him, and saw that the objects were starfish. "Why in the world are you throwing starfish into the water?" "If the starfish are still on the beach when the tide goes out and the sun rises high in the sky, they will die," replied the young man. "That's ridiculous. There are thousands of miles of beach and millions of starfish. You can't really believe that what you're doing could possibly make a difference!" The young man picked up another starfish, paused thoughtfully, and remarked as he tossed it out into the waves, "It makes a difference to this one."

Tonight I want one fellow-traveler, one caretaker of AIDS pilgrims, to know that you have made a difference.

In your willingness to be identified with those of us who live with too much stigma and die with too little grace; in your courage during times of uncertainty, your humor in times of despair, your affection when least we are lovable—in all this, you have become more than a beachcomber, more even than a caretaker. You have become a hero.

So here you are, God's angels and our heroes. Someday our children will sew you a quilt that remembers those who have served as surely as those who have died. Until then, God give you grace.

If I have come to embrace those who are HIV-positive, and encourage those who tend to our needs, then I have come to empower those of you who are our neighbors. You are the leaders of our community, the clergy in our houses of worship, the executives in our corporations, the presidents of our boards. You are students anticipating careers, parents raising our children, educators pursuing a better tomorrow for today's children. You are our neighbors.

Of all the groups here tonight, yours is the one I wish most I could reach. But the more I have spoken out over the past year, the less I am certain what to say. What must I do to move you?

Perhaps the young professionals among you would be moved by demographics. Does it bother you, for example, that by conservative estimates nine out of ten HIV-positive people in America have never been tested? They are "silently positive." They are here tonight. You might be one of them—if only once you had contact with someone who had contact with someone who had contact with someone who was "silently positive." If so, tomorrow you could go be tested. What holds you back is fear; you must be empowered. But I don't know how.

The truth is, I do not know what to say that will move my neighbors, young or old. Because I've found no way to convince you that you are at risk.

And what must I do to move those of you who love getting high? How can i explain that there is no one more at risk of HIV than the person who isn't sure what she did last night or with whom he left the bar? Getting high is the surest route to getting HIV. If I knew how to empower you, I would give you the gift of sobriety and give it early enough to save your life. But I don't know how.

The physical risk faced by all of those within the uninfected community is a virus. It's rampant, deadly, and avoidable. But there's another risk in our communities which is not physical; it is moral.

If you are a parent or a teacher, a pastor or a youth leader; if you have a position in which children or young adults model you—you manage moral risk. You determine whether stigma thrives in your home and classroom, or whether it dies. You set the patterns of intolerance or compassion, judgmentalism or grace. In your language, you teach respect or denigration. In your behavior, you set a model of charity or brutality. The more we have the capacity to lead in our homes, our houses of worship, our boardrooms and our classrooms, the more we will be held accountable for our communities' moral tone.

If I knew how to empower a community to avoid the risks, both physical and moral, I would do it gladly and often. But after a year of speeches, I am still searching for the right message to convince my neighbors, young and old, that you are even at risk.

And so, until you are convinced, I commend you to God's mercy, knowing nothing better to do.

Which leaves just one group among you, my family and my friends. When first I accepted this evening's engagement, I did not know you would be here. But you have honored me with your presence and I hope I've not bored you with mine. For those who have loved me most dearly, I have a simple request: Let us comfort one another. It's true that I'm not dying of AIDS, I'm living with HIV. But it's also true that death is a frequent caller among my fellow pilgrims. It's a context in which comfort can be as evasive as it is important.

Evenings at home with my children, we observe a bedtime ritual. As I tuck them in, I tell them to sleep with the angels. And then we say together the prayer which echoed through my childhood, as it probably echoed through yours:

> Now I lay me down to sleep,
> I pray the Lord my soul to keep . . . .

There have been hours when, since learning I am HIV-positive, I have been tired and ready to "lay me down to sleep." One grows weary of counting T-cells and telephone calls, of explaining it doesn't matter how one contracts this disease, of warning those who seem smugly content to ignore the warnings until their children take them aside and the family is shattered. I am grateful to you who have put your hands in mine and held me then. You've given me hope when mine slipped away, and lifted my spirits when I could not hoist them myself. You have come to me with comfort I could not find alone.

If, in the days of my anger at this virus, you heard only my cries of fear and frustration, diluted by no words of forgiveness and grace, then hear me tonight: The anger has already been eclipsed by commitment. And forgiveness, where it was needed, proved irresistible. If that is a comfort to you, hold it close.

Some here tonight have remembered the pain of death and loss. You've seen his face again, remembered his touch. You've bit your lip at the memory of her smile. You answered the call to courage, and still you weep at the message of forgiveness. I know. I weep too. Because the only path I know to comfort leads past a field of gravestones marking places they laid down to sleep.

But we who are here tonight, we have not yet laid down. We're able to make a commitment to those still walking and those who've stayed behind; and, in the morning, we're able to make a difference in our homes and schools and businesses and community. No matter what brought us here tonight, which group is ours, we could join a single, ragtag band of pilgrims in search of comfort.

I must leave, of course, but I would prefer not to go alone. I would miss the company of other pilgrims. And so to you, my friends and family, my neighbors and fellow-travelers, I issue a simple plea. Could we go together? The journey would be much sweeter, and our loads would be much lighter, if we could share them both.

Come, walk with me a little ways, seeking justice, fighting stigma, enjoying forgiveness, now and again, bending down to lift a starfish from the sand.

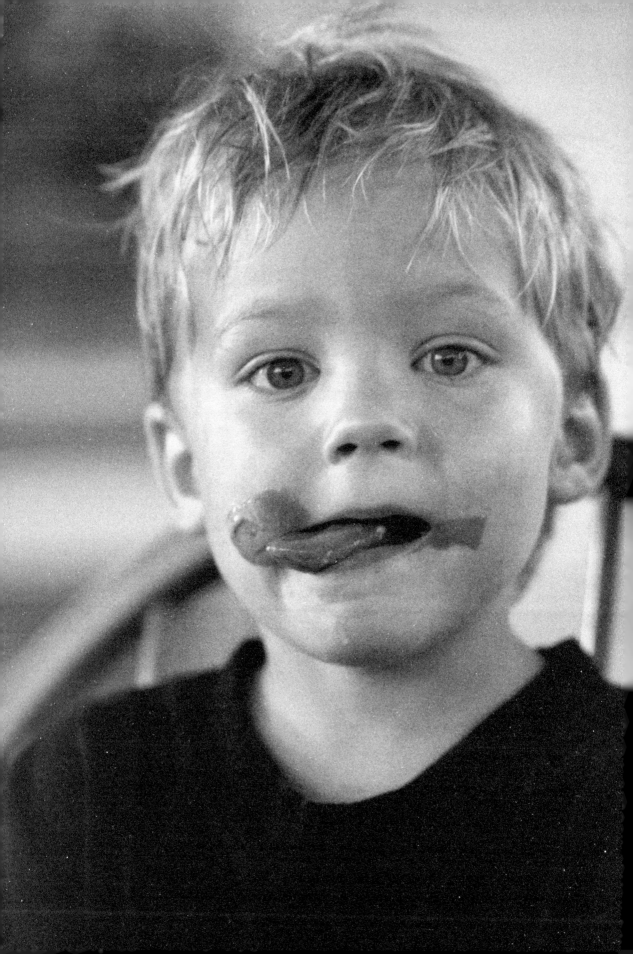

Publishing Courage

———————— o ————————

National Op-Ed Page Editors Conference
Detroit
April 18, 1993

Frank Bruni was the remarkable Detroit Free Press *reporter who, at editor Joe Stroud's behest, wrote the stories which broke the news that I was HIV-positive. Frank had, in the process, become a friend. And Joe Stroud had consistently offered to help in any way he could.*

Accepting the Free Press*'s invitation to address their conference for op-ed page editors from around the country gave me an opportunity to thank them publicly.*

But it also allowed me to speak candidly and personally to moral teachers in whose classroom every newspaper reader in America is already enrolled. These are the people who choose what will, and what will not, be printed. I was delighted to have dinner with them, and then to discuss the moral task that fills each of their working days.

I'd like to serve up a post-dinner menu of ideas in fairly brisk fashion, and see if any topics spark your interest or your questions. As speeches go, this one may have all the internal cohesion of a tossed salad. But it gives me a chance to offer a few private notions to a group of people who work under great public scrutiny.

Let me begin with a few personal notes.

First, as an HIV-positive person, it was rare good luck or pure grace that I chose to "go public" about my condition in *The Detroit Free Press* a little more than a year ago: February 1992. My family and I had wondered and worried and sometimes disagreed over my decision to tell my story publicly. When I indicated that I was going to tell my story first, here, in my hometown, in Joe Stroud's paper, I caused a level of consternation and anxiety among the Fishers which may have been unprecedented.

The story started on page one and rolled through the first section; television cameras watched the edition roll from the presses. It was more than we had expected, better than we had imagined, more worthwhile than I could have hoped.

But it wasn't me, or our family, that made it good. It was good, in part, because the *Free Press* assigned a young writer named Frank Bruni to do the story. He did it with a special blend of ingenuity, dignity, fairness and affection. To this day, more than a year later, I recall that story—and that man—with special gratitude.

And it was good because Joe Stroud has used his editor's pen to champion thoughtfulness and compassion in the face of an HIV/AIDS epidemic which has seen far too little of both. On more than one occasion, he has defended those who are HIV-positive and lifted up those who have fallen to AIDS. When mindless bigots have spewed ugly hatred, he has taken up his pen to call for decency. When critics said those who are HIV-positive deserve what they got, Joe Stroud wrote an editorial on the need for humanity in the wake of an inhumane illness. I'm glad I can be here tonight, Joe, to note publicly and with thanks your contribution to the struggle of more than a million-and-half or two million HIV-positive Americans and the twenty million people who live with and love them.

I am grateful for an opportunity to spend an evening in conversation with op-ed page editors of major newspapers. I don't know your personal histories. One episode from mine is centered around my decision to drop out of college—never to return, I might add—because I found the control room more attractive than the classroom. My first jobs in media were here, beginning at the local public television outlet and then becoming a full-fledged producer at Detroit's ABC owned-and-operated station. They were wonderful, dynamic years, full of joy and challenge and learning.

I learned then, and have not forgotten, the need for a good story. Reporting facts requires only a list; telling a story requires a plot. When a reporter or editor begins her or his interview with me, I'm sympathetic with their need for a story.

And editorial tasks are even more complicated. One must think and write not only clearly, not only for oneself, but persuasively and for an institution. Every day. Over and over and over again. When the dog days of summer drag on, the editorial gruel is thin; when the dogs of war howl and rage, the cost of a misjudged editorial may be your career.

Editors of op-ed pages, it seems to me, have a series of complicated and urgent mandates. You must find good issues, and then good ways to address them—but others' names must go under the material. Often, you devote a day to finding someone to disagree with you.

If morality is the consequence of making decisions reflecting our values, then your work is profoundly moral. You need to help sell the paper. But beyond that, you must judge what issues are sufficiently worthy to seduce the reader's attention as well as his coin. You need to decide when an opinion has been suffocated by too many words, or when it is being strangled by illogic. More importantly, you need to choose between those pieces or perspectives that are poignant, unusual, evocative and startling—and those which are mean, eccentric, dangerous and destructive. I admire the courage as well as the craft with which you must work.

You should know that I crisscross the nation telling people in HIV/ AIDS communities to work with their local media. I tell them they should not only write letters to the editor, they should get to know the editor, write op-ed pieces, and do what they can to influence editorial policies. I ask them how they expect editors and journalists to become sensitized without experience and without human relationships that make this issue tangible.

In fairness to them, let me render the same counsel to you. I wish you would be aggressive about seeking out people living with HIV in your community, and those who live with them. Get to know the parents who have lost a child, the orphans who are not yet able to ask the question, "Why?" Get to know the advocates, including those in organizations such as ACT-UP (which is by far more responsible and thoughtful than would be suggested by the coverage it has often attracted). Go into grade schools and high schools and colleges to ask what issues—including HIV- and AIDS-prevention—demand attention, and to invite youth participation in your pages—not just on the "youth page." Tell others to work with you. Get to know the caretakers and the care providers. Spend an hour in a hospice, if you haven't. It would be good not only for your soul but also for your art.

With due respect to the sensitivities many of you have no doubt honed to a fine edge, I am sometimes amazed at the insensitivity of editorial language when the topic is HIV and AIDS. When I am described as an "AIDS victim," I cringe. I am not a victim; nor, so help me God, do I ever intend to be one. I'm neither pathetic nor passive; I have been infected, not victimized. Similarly, I am not an "AIDS patient." I see my doctor about as often as most other women. On my doctor's charts, I may be a patient, but not on the pages of your newspaper. Like most others who are HIV-positive, I am a person living with the virus, not a victim or patient dying of it.

These are largely issues of sensitivity and choice. They can be dismissed, I suppose. The same thing happened when Martin Luther King argued against the use of the term "nigger" in Alabama in 1955. It's just a word. But words are the billboards of our souls, and its hard not to read through them.

To the extent that you play a critical role in setting your community's social, political, economic and moral agenda; and to the extent that your pages reflect your community's discussion of that agenda—to that extent, I hope you would seek to be both educated about this epidemic and sensitive to those who have been most captured by it.

It seems to me that the HIV/AIDS epidemic brings with it the problems that, from the perspective of editors, afflict many of the great crises. It is complicated and often ambiguous, wrapped up in a language which is inaccessible to the common person. It has a history which is largely subterranean and seldom well understood. The numbers are mindboggling and, therefore, mind-numbing. The best human interest stories can not be told for reasons of privacy. Side skirmishes—between fundamentalists ranting at one end and liberals screaming at the other— have limited shelf-life and even more limited editorial interest. And plaguing the whole thing is the need to find a new slant on a story or editorial position we feel we've run as often as a K-Mart ad. "How many AIDS babies pictures are worth printing?" we hardly dare ask out loud. *Gay Man Dies of AIDS-Related Causes* is not a stunning new headline. And how do we "cover" this epidemic without reinforcing stereo-types—of the sort leaping from that mythical headline?

I think my only response to this perennial issue—how one feeds a popular audience an unpopular diet of truth—is to urge that you not give up the effort.

The history of this epidemic is terribly important. In its history we discover that only in America is this seen as a "gay" disease. Here we learn that the rate of infections is one thing, and deaths resulting from AIDS are altogether different—and often divided by more than a decade. It's in the history of this epidemic that we come to understand the rage of gay activists and the terror of a single mother newly employed and now testing HIV-positive. It's in the history that we discover why we know almost nothing about HIV in women. I understand you are not history teachers; but I believe, unless you gain at least a passing familiarity with the history of this epidemic, you cannot adequately assess either its present course or its future trends.

Then there are the numbers. Big numbers. Huge numbers. Because epidemics start small and grow large, and because the span of time between infection and morbidity is so long, Americans are taking false security in reports of "AIDS deaths." Remember that those dying today were, in many instances, infected before we had yet coined the term "AIDS." If you want to grapple with numbers, grapple with the one-and-one-half or two million Americans like me who are HIV-positive with this one added fact: Approximately 90% of all HIV-positive are "silently positive"—they've never been tested. They don't know. Whatever it is that got them the virus is likely still occurring within their lives, thus making it a near certainty that they'll be passing it along. Now try your arithmetic.

And, as with all perennial issues faced in the newsroom or the editorial council, the haunting question becomes: How do we turn it into a story? I urge you, maybe I should beg you, to do this without flinching. When you finally lose your first friend to this disease, do not wait until you've stopped crying. Write your grief, and publish it. When you spend your hour in the AIDS hospice, write what it has done to you with your passion as well as with your pen. Don't sanitize this story with sterile facts. Let it be stained with human emotion. Nothing else will communicate the truth.

When you hear about a "cure," please be careful. Don't build false hopes in the minds of a few million parents and children. Or when you hear the prediction that this thing will never be cured, be careful how you handle the report. Living with HIV can be daunting, hope can be fragile, and suicide is no healthier an option than AIDS.

I cannot let go of the pain Arthur Ashe suffered because of an unwanted disclosure which reshaped the few remaining months of his life. No one meant to give him heart attacks. No one meant to give him AIDS. But someone *meant* to give him a headline. So many knew Arthur's condition: friends, physicians, fellow athletes—yes, and many journalists. But none felt the need to violate the man in the interest of a story. I wondered where that reporter was the afternoon of Arthur's funeral when one of the speakers—as it happens, it was Mayor Dinkens of New York—said: "In an age of better agents and better marketing, better releases and better images, here was, simply, a better man."

I must tell you that, almost without exception, I have been treated fairly and usually kindly by the press during the past year. Sometimes we've been amused by descriptions that are *overly* sympathetic or, worse yet, bordering on a kind of heroism one doesn't notice in a mirror.

But I worry that at least some of this treatment is coming at the expense of clear thinking and good moral sense. Here's my fear: I fear that stigma and bias have had their way, also with the media, and that I, Mary Fisher, am treated—as is Elizabeth Glaser, as was Ryan White, as was Arthur Ashe—as "an innocent in a field of guilt." Because I am straight, not gay; because I contracted the disease from a husband instead of a needle or a neighbor—therefore, the conception of this disease in my body was immaculate. And I am innocent.

To the extent that such thinking is having its way among those who shape public opinion, we should be terrified. It suggests that we withhold compassion from those whose behaviors may have caused or contributed to their deaths. On these grounds we would never mourn the passing of a heart attack victim who ate salt, worked under stress, or ate cholesterol. Persons with lung cancer owing to smoking should be disdained; persons with back injuries from lifting should be despised; the person who sees the ice but nonetheless slips on it should be left in agony where he landed. This is more than logically ridiculous. It is morally reprehensible.

Those who are quick to judge, who champion an arrogant morality which is more a weapon of attack than a call to decency—their voices are dangerous. And I hope you will never let them find expression without a challenge.

Compassion and dignity, justice and affection, these are the tools of morality with which we fight back in a battle against a virus which has, thus far, taken every person it ever visited.

To the extent that you wield those tools on an everyday basis, deciding which opinion should be heard and which should be muffled, I wish you great moral ambition and sturdy moral courage.

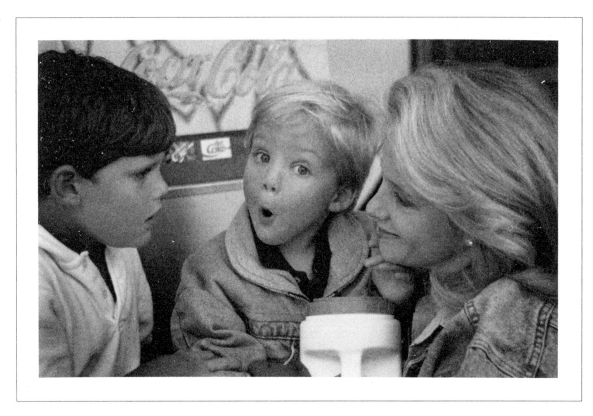

My Name Is Mary

———————O———————

Ecumenical AIDS Service, St. James Catholic Church
Grand Rapids, Michigan
April 22, 1993

If you've never attended a service in which those who've died of AIDS are being remembered, do. With one-and-a-half or two million HIV-positive Americans, and no cure, the opportunities for such services are multiplying in every community.

When people come to worship for the right reasons, they generate a power within the congregation which is unrivaled in any other setting. People of varying traditions are suddenly one; once we've all called God "Father," we are all brothers and sisters. And where else are we free to do in public all the things we do without embarrassment only when we are alone: sing, pray, shake our fists heavenward, ask "Why"? We are then free to sob in each other's arms.

Memorial services are, like the AIDS Quilt, all about names. We remember as the epidemic's toll mounts that it is not numbers who have died, but people. Each one has a name.

When, in the silence of the sanctuary, people softly say the names of those they are remembering, it is a time of wrenching sorrow. But it's the right place to bring this sorrow: into God's presence and into each other's arms and, therefore, into hope.

I have two names to which I respond. One is Mary. It's the name to which I've answered all my life—as a little girl, being called to dinner; as a young woman, answering the telephone, hoping for a Friday night date; as a professional woman, a married woman, an artist, a friend. It's a common name with an ordinary ring to it; fits me well. My name is Mary.

The other name to which I respond is "Mom." For more than five years now, it has been a name I first longed to hear, then thrilled to hear, and now, occasionally, grow weary of hearing. Of all my names, it is the one that never fails to remind me I am blessed, and loved. Whether it is five-year-old Max calling me to see his latest artwork, or three-year-old Zack prowling the kitchen to see where the cookies were hidden, they are God's best gifts to me. We're a family, my sons and I. And in our family, my name is "Mom."

It's true that I have a virus, and that the virus is deadly. But I am not a "patient" or a "case" for anyone. I do not focus on dying with this virus; I concentrate on living with it. I am, like you, a pilgrim stumbling along the way, a common pilgrim with a common name: Mary.

If you wish to be helpful you might remind me of who I am. Remind me that I am not a victim, that I want no pity. Remind me, with grace, that I am merely an ordinary person with an ordinary name: Mary.

Nearly two million Americans are HIV-positive; nearly two hundred thousand have already died in this epidemic. But I am not a statistic and I will never accept becoming one. I was not a number before learning my HIV status; I am not a number now. I am a person; I have a name. I am Mary.

Some of us have come tonight to grieve the loss of loved ones. We remember them with tears, we feel the aching lonesomeness that follows such loss. They are not numbers or statistics or victims to us. They are persons with names. Think of their names now. If you dare not say them aloud, whisper them softly to God. But if you can tell us, do. I've come remembering Kenn, and Alison, and John, and Belinda, and Arthur tonight. Tell me, any of you, what are the names of those you've lost?

We will remember them by their names.

Some have come tonight because you are HIV-positive. Some who know your name might be astounded to know your status. It does not matter. What matters is that you know that you are a person of infinite value, created by God and wrapped in grace. You are surrounded here tonight by people ready to love you. You have suffered enough. Continue to hide if you must, but ask for support if you can. Find a way to let us know and, in our hearts and our prayers, we will remember you by name.

If I could, tonight, I would offer healing and a cure. I would promise health; I would laugh at the virus and invite you to join in the laughter. But the healing I have to offer is prayer. The only cure, a family of people full of compassion, ready to love you cured or not. And for all, I have this promise.

God knows us by our names. Once, long ago, early on a Sunday morning, a grieving woman was moving toward a loved one's borrowed tomb. In the sunrise light she heard a voice, and then she heard him say, "Mary." He called her by her name—my name.

Those whom we've lost have not been lost by God; as surely as my children hear me calling "Max, Zack," they hear their Father calling them by name. Those who fear death, who dread illness, who suffer terror in the night: listen closely, and you will hear Him calling you—by your name.

As surely as he has drenched us in grace, he will give us comfort.

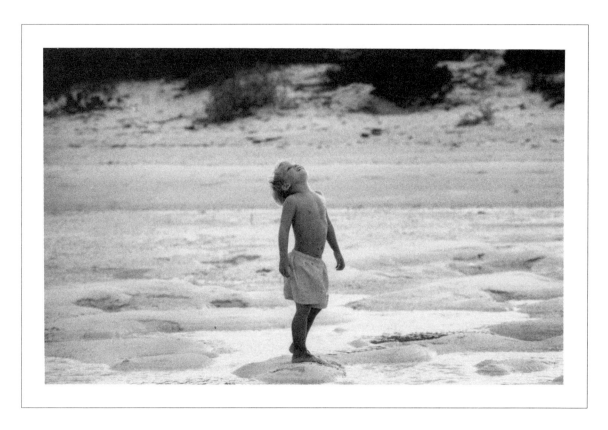

From One Commissioner's Chair

―――――――――― O ――――――――――

Cornell University Medical Center
New York City
April 29, 1993

*Dr. Henry Murray is Professor of Medicine at the Cornell
University Medical College and Chief of Infectious Diseases at
The New York Hospital, Cornell University. He's also my
"AIDS doctor" and a good friend.*

*Once each year the Medical Center has "Grand Rounds"
during which time hundreds of residents and physicians spend
a day in applied study together at the Center. This speech was
given, at Hank's request, at the conclusion of 1993 Grand
Rounds.*

*Members of the AIDS community depend on the medical
community for life itself. Members of the medical community
are growing frustrated with AIDS because it does not let them
do what most they want to do: heal. There is currently no cure.
And until a cure is found, we need ways to keep the medical*

community fully engaged in this epidemic.

But no one needs to help Hank Murray. He's fully engaged, and it shows. No one wept harder when Arthur died than Hank, who had tried so hard to keep him alive another day.

Epidemics can no more escape history than can people. The impact of the early context of AIDS within gay communities has had enduring consequences. Because the epidemic broke first among gay men, research priorities were shaped to men, not women. When the virus jumped over the gender fence, we had little to no information regarding HIV in women.

Because gay and lesbian communities have been politically volatile, the epidemic itself was politicized from the very beginning. Since the politics affecting AIDS issues was a politics of polarization, no majority has emerged with a commonly accepted agenda and venue.

Because the virus was attached to "being gay" or "being promiscuous"—or, later, to being a "drug abuser"—those who are infected have feared disclosure. Patterns of denial emerged, both in those who are infected and those around them, which have made reasonable, public health responses difficult or impossible.

And because all of these consequences can be debated in moral terms, AIDS has become a battleground for the politics of morality from the small-town pulpit to the United States Senate. Listen to debates on immigration or research funding, and you'll hear the concept of common decency taking a beating.

It's imperative that we recognize the tremendous impact cultural history has had on this particular epidemic. When we lose sight of these realities, we are condemned to failure.

This is an epidemic whose institutional response is essentially leaderless. During early days, institutions rose within the gay communities which were "community-based organizations" with a local focus.

Then came the American Foundation for AIDS Research (AmFAR) which—founded in part by Elizabeth Taylor because of Rock Hudson—added a certain star quality to the epidemic. But no single institution has taken the leadership role. The federal government has been paralyzed, largely by the politics discussed a moment ago. The scientific community has been underfunded and overly segmented. The social, cultural, and religious communities have been unwilling to go to the front in this war. Even recommendations of the National Commission on AIDS, on which I sit, have had no noticeable effect on either the previous or the current Administration. There simply is no single leader here. As a result, institutions are competing with each other for talent, for funds, for political clout and national prestige. The quality of institutions which are in the hunt for leadership perks and funding dollars varies widely, and there is no impartial body to tell the truth to the public. The infected community is itself deeply divided along cultural, ethnic and economic lines; and because there's no single, trusted voice in this arena, the mythology which has grown up with AIDS is persistent. AIDS is really two epidemics: one caused by a virus, the other by mistrust and confusion.

In the absence of leadership, the epidemic is clearly winning the upper hand.

If you wanted to design the epidemic that would ruin the fragile systems now in place, AIDS would be the near-perfect instrument of destruction. It strikes those who would otherwise not be major clients of the system: the young, in the prime of their lives. It follows routes of transmission that bring it disproportionately to communities of color and of poverty. Where young mothers are at risk, they are often infected; where they are infected, at least a third of their children are infected. The disease itself requires years of extended treatment which grow increasingly more intense and most costly. Absence of either an effective preventative or a reliable cure tends to make the disease itself a demoralizer for healthcare professionals. Insurance companies will look for routes out of responsibility at the same time the ordinary course of the disease requires extended, inpatient care. Give this epidemic a good head start so that, let's say, we get at least a million or two infections around the country, and we add significantly to the stress on the healthcare system in major metropolitan areas like New York in the immediate future.

Given the historical context of AIDS, the lack of leadership in our response to it and the threat it poses to the healthcare system, what kind of response is needed? Let me quickly summarize three responses that I believe are urgent.

First, a public-private response is imperative. This epidemic is simply overwhelming to both government and the private sector. A partnership isn't a nice idea; it's an imperative action. And at least to date, it hasn't captured the imagination of either sector.

I have consistently argued that, if we're to win this battle, everyone needs to do what they do best—and this extends to institutions as well as individuals.

The government is not a good leader, because it is directed by politicians who follow their constituency—they almost never actually lead anyone anywhere. If there is going to be a leadership group, therefore, it must be drawn at least largely from the private sector. Thus far, it has not emerged.

The government is historically better at stimulating the private sector to meet national priorities than it is at meeting them itself. For example, during World War II the government quickly abandoned its plan to produce armaments and weapons of war, providing profits instead to the private sector which converted auto plants to tank plants and petroleum refineries to munitions plants. In the battle with AIDS, the government could take such steps as insuring tremendous tax breaks to pharmaceutical firms—even a dollar-for-dollar corporate tax rebate for AIDS-directed research. To date, no such stimulus has found its way to the floor of Congress.

We need a national "management information system" which will immediately network all researchers; it can only work through a dynamic, well-funded private-public partnership. Here and there the elements of this system have been forged; overall, it is still lacking.

And there is no national leadership voice. No matter what your political persuasion, the voice of C. Everett Koop was important on the issue of smoking. We lack such a voice today. Without it, I doubt that we will achieve an effective private-public partnership, because there is no one to call the parties to the table.

A second ingredient in healthcare response is training for healthcare providers. Here, as today is a witness, we may be gaining ground. Physicians and other healthcare providers are as subject to mythology and prejudice as anyone, and it is especially critical that they not succumb.

When, about a year ago, a professional woman friend of mine asked her OB/GYN for an HIV test, he told her it wasn't necessary because she wasn't "that kind of woman." That gentleman's ignorance is dangerous; his knowledge of science may have been adequate, but his capacity for sensitivity was grossly inadequate. I would hope instead for physicians who have no desire to hide either ignorance or emotion behind white coats. In the absence of a cure, I would hope for compassion. Beyond that, I would hope for a senior doctor's encouragement to a young researcher to think about AIDS, and a consulting physician's guidance so a medical team incorporates the patient as its most critical member. Before healthcare providers establish their professional credentials, they need—to be helpful with those facing AIDS—to establish their credentials as human beings: as a father or mother, brother or sister, lover or friend.

Therefore, I welcome today's opportunity to raise our awareness to the realities of this epidemic—and I pray for the day that medical schools, nurses' training programs, and continuing-education programs across the nation will increase knowledge, sensitivity and interest that will help close the chapter on AIDS.

Finally, I'd appeal to each of you to become part of the leadership within your local communities. Children and teenagers listen to physicians in a way that they will not listen to parents or teachers. If you are a physician *and* a parent, you already know which role gives you the most status. I must tell you that some months ago I visited Hank Murray's daughter's school, and the fact that Hank took time out—not once, but twice—to visit first with the students and then with the parents, made our time there much more valuable than I could have made it alone.

Women's groups in your community, especially those affiliated with such organizations as the YWCA, need help. And the clergy in most communities would respond much more quickly to a call from a group of local physicians than to a call from, say, Planned Parenthood.

You've earned, with your rigorous training and historic role in America's healthcare system, a position of trust and leadership which could make a great difference in our fight. I was, myself, brought into the battle quite against my own will. But if I was drafted, you could enlist—and all of us, including me and my children, could certainly use your help.

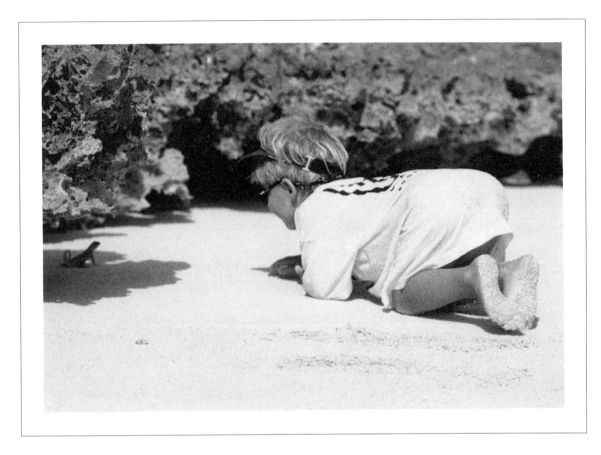

As You Pass By

————————o————————

Trinity College Commencement
Hartford, Connecticut
May 23, 1993

When Trinity College called to say they would like to award me an honorary degree—a doctorate, a Ph.D. yet!—and then have me address their graduating class, I was stunned. And elated. I gave it serious thought and, three seconds later, accepted.

And the event itself was exactly what I'd imagined it would be: full of tradition and academic ceremony, crowds of graduates and parents, clean-shaven administrators and bearded faculty, caps and gowns and "Pomp and Circumstance." And—would my parents ever believe this?—me: the commencement speaker at historic Trinity College.

Today marks the one hundred sixty seventh time this extraordinary college community has gathered to congratulate and wish God's speed to its graduates. My congratulations to you, the members of the Class of 1993. I am honored that you asked me to join you, and even to speak to you, on this occasion. I was especially humbled that you would give me, by grace, what you—and my sister Margie—spent years earning with clenched-jaw determination: a degree from Trinity College.

Mark Twain, writing from a home not far from here, urged us to tell the truth because, he said, "it will confound your enemies and amaze your friends." Receiving a doctorate has approximately the same effect in my life. I have only two regrets: One, that my parents—who previously had a dropout and now have a doctor in the family—were not here to be amazed in person. And, two, that a certain professor from a great, midwestern university—who so greatly contributed to my drop-out status—could not be here to be confounded.

Together with others, you have honored me today. We are all grateful. But we do not want you to follow us with imitation; we want, sometimes desperately, for you to pass us by and keep going. The study you've completed and the degree you've earned, both prove that you are competent to pass us by. But what you've now achieved in college must, if you are to make a difference in life, be matched by achievements in character.

I know that you are on the road to success in America; you know that I am on the road to AIDS. But did you know that, fundamentally, it does not matter? Both roads will end at the same place. And along the road, if we are remarkably gifted, we will discover a simple truth: that the length of our life is less important than its depth.

Americans are obsessed with making their lives long; we would do better if we put at least equal energy into making our lives valuable.

Americans are obsessed with achievement, with competence. Your degree is proof that you have already passed the test of compe-tence. That's good. But what lies ahead is a lifetime in which you not only may, but certainly will, prove your character. And it is character that will ultimately determine whether you are just another tourist ambling down life's road, or whether you are a pilgrim whose eyes are riveted on the goal and whose journey itself is a testimony to grace.

If I knew this truth before two years ago, I did not know it as I know it now. In this regard, the virus which I detest has refocused my life in unexpected, and unwanted, and wonderful ways.

Once I thought of wisdom as "having all the answers." I no longer hold that view. Looking at my sons—Max, who's five, and Zachary, who's three—I realize that I don't care if, when they are grown, they've mastered all the answers. Because life will bring them questions for which no answer has been devised. What I pray for them, and for myself, and now for you, is *wisdom*, the ability to live by trust when we have no answers.

I have always been a person of organization and order. I despise confusion and uncertainty. I like schedules kept and projects completed. I like control over my life. And into my life has come a tiny virus to teach me, again, that I am not in control. I can respond by giving up hope and embracing despair, by whimpering and retreating. Or I can cling to my conviction that in all things there is good purpose. And, in that conviction, I might live wisely—by trust—while I have no easy answers.

The power of death is enormous, and the bloodiness which results from evil is staggering. How long did it take for us to go from Hitler's "final solution" to today's "ethnic cleansing"?

In general, of course, we know how to satisfy questions such as, "How long has it been?" But when we come to the question, "Why?" we discover that there are few satisfying answers. The issues are not merely personal, or psychological. They are broad and tough. How do we, who are African-Americans, live with confidence when we still hear auctioneers and rattling chains in the night? How do we, who are women, choke back anger and press forward with courage in a culture that warns us to keep our place? How do we, who are Jewish, hold onto faith when we smell smoke pouring from the ovens? How do we who are gay keep the will to survive? And why? Why must good women and men struggle against evil? Why must pilgrims bleed?

Such questions will help us stay awake at night. They'll teach us how few satisfying answers we have. But if we are wise, we can trade sleeplessness for comfort. Because wisdom is not the ability to field every question; it is the capacity to live life, joyfully, when we have no answers.

In the end, wisdom will shape our view of life itself. If it is true that we are, all of us, pilgrims on the road, then it is wisdom that teaches us how to value this life, this journey.

Look at you: bright and beautiful, educated and eager, full of life and ready to throw mortar boards high enough to tease the angels. What a thrilling sight you are.

And I am no less encouraged when, not as a speaker but as a pilgrim, I look back on the road we are traveling and see you coming up behind me. If some in the marketplace would see you as a crowd of competition, I see you as a growing community of comfort.

Perhaps from the Class of '93 will come the philosopher who helps answer the great "Whys" of life, the musician or the poet who will teach us the sounds of peace, the researcher who will find the cure. You who seize not only an education, but also wisdom, will come down the road as a company of courage—not lacking fear, but acting wisely when most you are afraid.

I have two prayers for you. The first is a hard prayer for a commencement celebration, but I would have no integrity if I did not offer it today. It is my prayer that you will know your own mortality, that you will know the reality of your death before you set out on the rest of your life.

This is not a depressing vision of the Grim Reaper standing over you, ready to snatch you from life. It is merely the gift that came hard to me. In facing the reality that I cannot hoard my own life, store it up and save it, I discovered the extraordinary delight in giving it away. And it is that gift I pray for you.

I do not know how many women and men, famous and wealthy, have come to the end of their lives only to discover that they are bitterly unhappy. They have taken their wonderful inheritance and their decorated degrees, and devoted their lives to gathering riches and reputations and rewards. And then, at the end of their lives, they look back on the wreckage of their own values. When the fever jumps, they would trade their stock portfolio in an instant for the cooling kiss of a child they no longer know. What they miss is not the sound of applause, but the quiet murmur of a lover and friend. Too late, they discover the value of love.

It is hard reality, not fragile romance, that drives me to this prayer: May you grasp your own mortality early in your life. Because pilgrims who cherish their journey do it with love. They are the ones who have learned not to hold back when a parent needs to know her value in their lives. They are the ones with courage enough to risk heartbreak in family and friendships, because they have learned that love is the art of giving ourselves to others—without worrying about what will be given in return.

And my second prayer for the Class of '93 is one of gratitude. Knowing that you are on the road behind me gives me great hope. When I see you coming toward me, from the distance, I take new courage. Because sometimes I am not as wise as I should be. Lacking answers to hard questions, I grow frightened. Looking into the future, I worry that I will grow weary, and not be able to go on. For myself, I would be happy enough for a rest, but my children. . . .

And then I see God's company of comfort—you—coming up behind me. And I say to myself, "They will be wise, and come with joy. They will be loving, and come with charity." Don't you see, that is why you are my company of comfort?

If your parents must age and your professors must retire—if we, who are the pilgrims ahead of you, must lie down for a while, it is all right. Because here you come, our company of comfort!

You are our comfort because we are convinced that when you hear the echoes of slavery, the whispers of discrimination; when you feel the heat of the ovens of hatred, kindling new reasons for evil and death; when you see those who are ill cowering under moral judgment, those who are gay being battered with bigotry—we take our comfort in the conviction that you will rise up to say, "No more!"

You are my company of comfort because I know that, as you pass me by, you will sweep up my children in your arms and carry them on with you. And so, you will give me reason for great joy and sweet comfort.

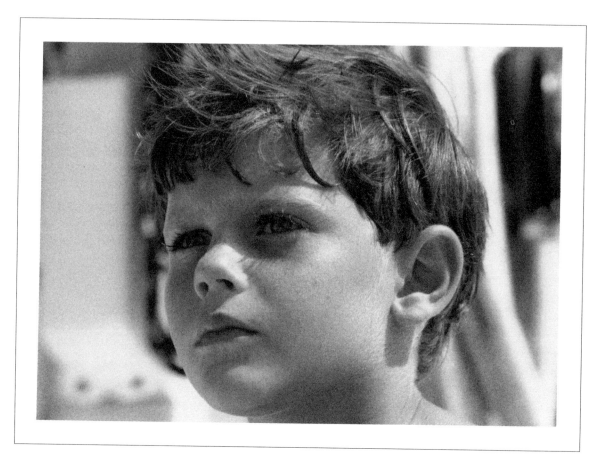

Come, Dream with Me

---O---

Mamaroneck High School
Mamaroneck, New York
June 7, 1993

Speaking to high school students—which I've done across the country—is, for me, an unequal exchange. They get a little of my time and I get a lot of their love.

The formal speeches themselves are often as much for the faculty and administration, the counselors and visiting parents (and media), as for the students themselves. In reality, I have nothing to tell young adults that I don't also want to say to their parents and grandparents.

It's what happens after the formal speeches that make these extraordinary events. When I leave the stage and walk into the audience to explain how we don't get AIDS, and ask if someone would risk touching me, an emotional dam breaks and we become bonded—a crowd of boisterous teenagers and a forty something mother of two.

181

In the moments following high school speeches I've had juvenile offenders, brought in by the sheriff, ask if they could have a hug before returning to custody. I've had a faculty member work his way through a churning crowd of his own students to take my hands, whisper "I'm a pastor who believes in healing," and pray that God will make me whole. I've heard teenagers confess their own terror of being at risk, their uncertainty of how to be tested, their fear of talking to their parents. I've heard a terrified young man blurt out, "I tested positive. . .don't tell anybody." And, countless times, "My uncle died of AIDS, and my parents won't let me talk about it."

This speech was given in Mamaroneck, New York. It could have been given in almost any junior or senior high school in America.

In many high school assemblies about AIDS, the speakers are athletes. Magic Johnson, for example, often visits colleges and schools. And talking about Magic may be a good place for me to begin my own story with you, because Magic may be the person who most inspired me to go public about being HIV-positive.

The story really begins in the summer of 1991, almost two years ago. I'd recently been divorced and was, as we like to say, "getting my act together." I was enjoying my work as a professional artist. And, as a young mom, I was taking special joy in my two sons: Max, who was then three, and Zachary who was just one. Life was in a pretty good place.

Then came a telephone call from my ex-husband saying he'd tested positive for the AIDS virus. I was tested within hours, but it took two weeks to get the results. The rest of that summer, and the months stretching toward the winter holidays, were grim. I was really uncertain how best to respond to this new situation when one November day I joined the rest of America, watching Magic's smile dance across a news conference in which he described AIDS as a challenge to be faced, something to be lived with. I caught a vision of hope that afternoon that has never fully faded—and, as Magic knows, I'm grateful to him.

Arthur Ashe was also important to my life. When you think of American athletes and AIDS, the names of Magic and Arthur are quick to be mentioned. A name not especially linked to this epidemic is that of Manute Bol, the seven foot seven inch basketball phenomenon who was born and raised in the Sudan of Africa. A just-released book tells the remarkable life story of Manute Bol, a giant in a land of famine. It's a wonderful book about values and priorities. In it, there's a scene in which Manute has returned to the Sudan and seen the hunger of his homeland. He's measured his life in America with all its splendor and fame. And he murmurs out loud, "I wonder what God is dreaming for us."

I've wondered that myself in the past two years. I believe that in all things there is a good purpose; hearing my children laugh, watching them sleep quietly in the night, I wonder what the good purpose may be in this virus.

It's hard to find a good purpose in a withering epidemic which has already taken two hundred thousand lives in America alone. It's not clear what God is dreaming for us when we begin to count the numbers: One-and-a-half or two million Americans like me, already infected with HIV—soon to be AIDS.

It's not even clear to me what I should be doing about it. I've spoken to audiences from New York to Los Angeles. You can imagine what I've hoped to do: I've tried to keep others from becoming infected. I've wanted to leave my children a legacy of decency and perhaps even courage, so that one day they will look back and know that their mother was no victim and no coward. To say it simply, I've wanted to make a difference in lives like yours.

But I don't know how. The more I've spoken out over the past year, the less I'm certain what I must say. What must I do to move you? What must I say, or demonstrate, or prove that would stir you to action? What words could effectively challenge either your denial or your confidence that, just as *I* was never at risk, neither are you?

I've heard that some people find the idea of abstinence amusing. But I've noticed that very few find the idea amusing at a moment like this. Because only those here this morning who have been absolutely abstinent, or who had no blood transfusion before the mid-1980s, is beyond the pool of risk. So far. For the rest of us, the edge of fear that grips our stomach is justified.

If I knew how, I would take each of you who has already put yourself at risk for an HIV test. It could set your mind at ease, or it could confirm your fear—but at least it would equip you to extend your own life and save the lives of others. And if I knew how, I would find the words that could keep you from further risk. But I just don't know what words those are.

Does it make a difference if I remind you, for example, that during the past two years the number of teens and young adults diagnosed with AIDS increased by 77 percent? But it can't be you, can it? Because anyone with whom you would have a relationship isn't "that kind of person." It's amazing to me, because I'm not "that kind of person" either.

By twelfth grade, according to national statistics, three-fourths of all students have had sexual intercourse and 19% of all high school students report having four or more sex partners. That's a terrifying piece of information to me. And I don't know what to do about that, or about this: Of sexually active high school students, less than half report that they or their partners have used a condom. Maybe you can tell me later how this can be changed.

And if there's anyone here who believes AIDS belongs in dirty city streets—that we are saved by geography—let me bother you with just one more number: Already years ago, the spread from city to suburb was underway. In 1990, AIDS cases actually grew seven times faster in the suburbs than in the cities.

If I knew how to empower you with self-discipline, with the sense of self-esteem and affection that makes abstinence possible, I would give it to you in an instant. If I knew how to empower you with the gift of sobriety and clear thinking, and to give you these gifts early enough to save your life, I'd do it in an instant. If only I knew how.

I have three requests of you.

First, I wish you would commit yourselves to a campaign for compassion. Since the earliest days of this epidemic in America, when AIDS was first identified with the gay male population, this has been an epidemic marked by stigma, discrimination, and cruelty. We have isolated persons who are HIV-positive. We have driven little children from classrooms and whole families from neighborhoods. We have let ignorance and fear take the place of knowledge and courage. We have written, as a nation, a history of shame—not for those who are HIV-positive, but for those of us who slandered and persecuted them. From locker-room humor which cuts until we bleed, to self-righteous moral judgments which mock the call to compassion, our national response to this epidemic has been marked by abuse.

Most of you are at an age where I cannot hold you responsible for our past, and I don't. But I, and history itself, will hold you responsible for the choice you make now and in the future: Either you will join those who have championed oppression or you will enlist in the fight against it. You will make your own choices on whether to tell the cruel joke, or withhold it; whether to point fingers and wag your head at those who struggle with AIDS, or whether to reach out and lift their burdens. You can ask your parents to speak with compassion, or you can sit idly by.

I am asking you, today, to move toward compassion. To seek justice. To demand decency in care and treatment of those who are sick and dying. I will not accept as an excuse that you are too young; that's nonsense. If on a football field you are capable of attracting the attention of tens of thousands of people, including adults of all ages, then in a struggle between life and death you are capable of making a good moral choice.

My second request is that you act on that compassion. What kind of action would that require? Well, at a minimum, you'd not put yourself at risk. You'd not seduce others to risk, either.

Beyond that, you would become involved. If you have the ability to teach, teach those who are younger than you. Go into Sunday School classrooms and grade school playgrounds, to encourage those who admire you. Go into your little sister's bedroom and tell her, in language and ways that are appropriate for her age, that you love her enough to value her life—and you want her not to squander it. Show your little brother that you could be a model worthy of following; break through the macho image long enough to say, "It's hard to make all the right choices, but if we love each other, we can help each other do it."

Talk to your parents, if they haven't spoken to you. Parents suffer a strange affliction: They don't dare talk unless they believe they have all the answers. No one has all the answers about AIDS; if they did, I wouldn't be here. So *you* start the conversation with your parents. Ask what they know, or would like to know. See if they are living with a silent terror which could be lifted in a quiet conversation with you. Be willing to break down hard barriers with a single soft phrase: "I love you. . . ."

And if you have a moment of time, and a heart touched by grace, then go to work in the community. Volunteer an hour or two at your local AIDS centers. Visit a hospice and see if there's a time you could read a book to someone who has lost his eyesight to AIDS. Break out of a safe and contented world dominated by self-fulfillment to touch, and be touched, by an epidemic which is unavoidable.

That is my second request. And my third is very simple. It has to do with my children. It is my prayer that I will see them grow to your age, and beyond. But I have less certainty than most parents. I make no assumptions any more about the length of my life.

And so, sometimes when I am wondering what God is dreaming for us, I wonder what kind of world you will help shape for my children. You will be entering leadership roles in life as my children enter high school. You will be helping to set the moral tone in America, the national priorities, the agenda which my children will follow.

My final request to you is this: Please do better for my children than my generation did for you. We sacrificed a good deal on the altar of financial success, often turning too quickly from our children to balance our checkbooks. Some of us adults, who take such pride in our homes and businesses, and even in our terribly public acts of public charity, have no relationships left in our homes which are worthy of pride. And you who are sitting with me this morning suffer it. You hear the raging battles between your parents and you wonder if you'll be the first to leave, or if one of them will. You feel the anger of a woman who wishes she'd not given up a career, and you feel guilty. You see too many drinks going down a father's throat, and you imagine that he's swallowing too much emotion. I know. These are the hard realities we try to gloss over with a heroic image, a Friday night beer or two, and the behaviors which could cost you your life. But, please, don't. Succeed where some of us have failed. Set a standard which my children could see, a standard that calls for charity in the place of judgment. Imitate the acts of compassion which mark the best of us, rather than the worst.

I don't know what God is dreaming for us, exactly. But in the quiet moments of the night when my children are finally asleep, and I turn to rest for a little while, I sometimes take comfort in the knowledge that compassion can conquer what even science cannot understand.

I'm grateful you are here, that you are within a moment's decision to save your own life, and that you have the power to choose compassion. And I'm sorry that I must go. But when I leave, I would like to take with me your commitment to the struggle. Come with me, if you would, to the promise of compassion and courage. Come say a word to me, if you wish, or give a hug. Come dream with me, until we wake to joy and hope.

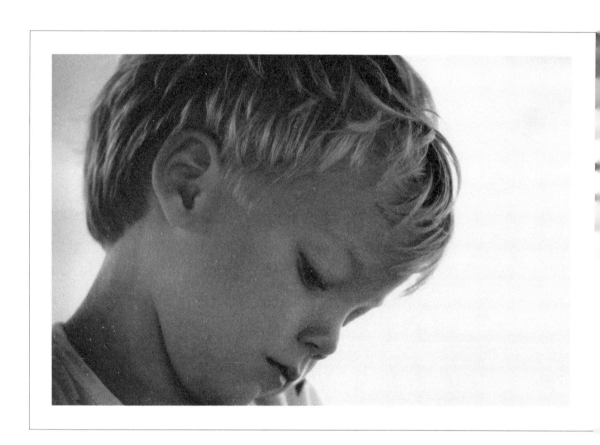

When Pilgrims Stumble

———————O———————

78th Annual Catholic Health Association Membership Assembly
1993 Father John J. Flanagan Lecture
New Orleans, June 8, 1993

Catholics, Protestants, Jews, Muslims—we all tend to imagine that we are different from others. Perhaps we are, at least in some of the particulars. But in our search for God, we become amazingly similar to one another, common pilgrims who walk a common path.

I remember talking about this to the crowd in the huge New Orleans ballroom. Gigantic screens had been mounted on either side of the podium where I spoke, enabling the audience to see me larger-than-life. I thought there were too many of me.

But it was a responsive audience, quick to laugh and unafraid of tears—good people who did not have a hard time understanding that all of us who are pilgrims will, from time to time, stumble.

It's a pleasure to be here today for a number of reasons, but two are probably self-evident: I'm glad to speak to an audience which is composed largely of caregivers, and I'm glad to speak to an audience which is composed largely of Catholics, or at least Catholic sympathizers—among whom I would number myself.

One evening last August I gave a brief speech to some politically minded folks who had gathered in Houston. It was a minority group of sorts; they called themselves "Republicans."

By profession I am not a public speaker. By interest and training, I am an artist. By grace, I am a mother. These two callings, artist and mother, consume and renew my life with joy and challenge and contentment. In general, these are the only two careers which I confess to holding. Which is to say, I am not a politician. And neither am I a theologian, a fact which some members in your respective traditions would say uniquely qualifies me to speak to a group of you.

I was raised in a Jewish home by parents who are spiritually sensitive. My mother, especially, has devoted a good deal of her adult life to spiritual exploration into some interesting territory. But I was a bit taken back last fall when, as part of a speaking tour in the Carolinas, I was invited to deliver a sermon in a large Presbyterian church. I wasn't sure I was qualified, but I tackled it anyway.

As with the first disciples, word soon got out. I received other invitations—and accepted them—to preach in other congregations, from the Carolinas to California. Each time I mounted a new pulpit, I was welcomed and introduced as an honorary member of the faith. Therefore, while I have no formal theological training, I come to you this afternoon as America's only Episcopalian Presbyterian Catholic Baptist Jewish woman. . .who's an HIV-positive Republican.

Just before Easter I was in Texas for a meeting of the National Commission on AIDS. A friend in California, who'd heard me preach there, sent a copy of my sermon to his friend, the senior pastor of perhaps the largest Southern Baptist congregation in Texas. And so I was invited to address *that* congregation. I arrived at the church with little time to spare but was warmly welcomed by the senior pastor. We spoke for just a few moments while heading toward the pulpit together. Just before entering the sanctuary, he asked about my "home church." I said, "Ah, home temple—I'm Jewish."

He stopped breathing just as I mounted the pulpit. Not knowing what else to do, I left him for dead. But there he was when I'd finished, alive and well, smiling, greeting his congregation. Raised in a Jewish context, it was the sort of experience that gives me new appreciation for the Christian doctrine of the resurrection.

I presume that many of you here embrace that resurrection as a critical component not only of your faith, but also of your caregiving. The earliest Christian-Jewish communities lived in a context of the Roman Empire where deformed children were despised; so despised, in fact, that they were brought to the hillsides and left to die. There, under cover of darkness, the early church sent its deacons to rescue the children. It's no wonder that when St. Paul speaks of our union with God, he speaks of it as an adoption. In the Christian tradition, one gives care not for money nor for self-advancement, not for a Mercedes or a government grant, but for God.

I commend you for that tradition. And much of what I have to say this afternoon is rooted in my conviction that if that tradition could take wings and fly across America today, the AIDS community in this nation would be instantly and vastly improved.

When I think of the millions already infected with the AIDS virus—including at least one-and-a-half or two-million Americans—I think of them as a great, long band of pilgrims. I visualize that band as a ragtag army of people drawn from every race and tribe, color and character. It is not a parade of wealth or privilege. It is not a march led by shining trumpets and dancing drummers. It is not a crowd of the world's powerful. It is a barefooted, dusty crowd whose edges are crowded and whose organization is uncertain. It's a crowd of persons inclined more to look down than to look up, despite the fact that these pilgrims are proud; more prone to silence than to shouting; a band of young who look old, of people grown weak but still lifting the children onto their shoulders; a slowly moving river of people. I think of them as pilgrims.

The Catholic tradition contains the story of Father Damien's missions to the leper colonies of Hawaii and beyond. I was once told that Father Damien had preached many a strong sermon of hope and courage in those colonies before the Sunday morning when his homily took special meaning. "They never heard the gospel," he recalled, "until that morning." It was the sun-drenched day he turned to his leprous congregation and began, "We lepers. . . ."

I've used the pilgrim band metaphor in every public speech I've given for some months. I do it consciously, and I'd like you to know why.

I want those who are HIV-positive to think of themselves as moving not only toward AIDS but also toward God. I want the historic imagery of Bunyan's pilgrim making progress to show character in the making, to reveal our life as filled with purpose and promise.

I want those who are HIV-positive, and especially those who care for them—the physicians and parents, nurses and nuns, lovers and strangers—to know that they become witnesses to others whenever they become part of the public pilgrimage. It takes courage to admit to ourselves that we are HIV-positive. It takes double courage to tell others. Therefore, when those infected and those who love them join the public march, they are giving testimony simply by walking with us.

I want those who are quick to judge the HIV-positive pilgrims to know that they are pilgrims, even when they are no longer humble or contrite. When they are angry young men losing weight and losing life, howling in rage and hurling condoms at the passing limousines, they are still pilgrims. When they are prostitutes slinking out of sight or infants gasping for breath; playwrights penning stunning dramas or dancers twisting in the air; gay couples flaunting their choices or grief-stricken mothers tucking their children into bed; homeless women too sick to care or priests who still deliver their homilies—these are not objects of pity; these are human beings shaped in God's image, moving toward God's future, pilgrims.

And I refer to the AIDS community as a pilgrim band *in part* as a reproach to the religious community in America. The images and metaphors which have been used as brands to mark people in the AIDS community—since the earliest days, when the illness began destroying gay communities—have often reflected moral and religious stereotypes that are unworthy of our great religious traditions. In some small way I want to challenge and change that image. And so I've adopted the vision of a pilgrim band. I am convinced that in the sweep of human history, God is at work also through the AIDS community of which I am a part. Therefore, we are not merely infected; we are called.

Spirituality has been a very important part of my life for some time. It is not a new caller who met me after I learned I was HIV-positive. In fact, I think I've never been in a more spiritually centered place than I was the month I discovered that the virus had found me.

My own sense of the reality of God, of my connectedness to all of creation, has been the source of great security in my life. Within days of hearing the test results and knowing that I was on the road to AIDS, I told a close friend that I *knew* that in all things there was a divine purpose. It took me some months to begin sensing what that purpose might be in my life, but—apart from the darkest hours when all faith scattered—I did not doubt that there was a purpose and a calling.

It's terribly important that you who are leaders in religious healthcare hear this story, not because it is my story but because, in many respects, it is yours. You are the ones who call for faith, even when your own is fragile. You are pressed to give answers of certainty, even when you are uncertain; to offer prayers, even when you doubt the value of prayer. You are the ones who must blow softly on the embers of ancient traditions to bring them newly to life in modern moments, wondering, all the while, if it matters.

When I asked wise and trusted friends what I could do to support the pilgrim band, they consistently told me the same thing: "Tell your story in public." And so I have. Today, part of the story I want you to hear is that faith made a difference. It helped carry me over tortuous territory in those first, staggered days. It nudged me past incredible terrors and stunning depressions. It encouraged me to seek not pity but purpose. It reminded me that I am not the Giver or Keeper of my life, and that I cannot save it; therefore, I would be wise to give it away before it is squandered. Faith made a difference.

And, therefore, I have this message for you and your institution: Because faith matters, you matter. In the face of political and cultural stigma, your insistence that God loves justice, it matters. Your insistence that in all things there is God's handiwork, that the whisper of comfort drifting over the pilgrim band is God's voice, it matters.

My confidence that God is central enabled me, early on, to know that there is a "bigger picture" than Mary Fisher and her children and her home and her life. My conviction that God pours life through us to others, so that it flows again toward God, reminds me to stay focused away from myself. I find it a great relief to know that I am not indispensable; how else could I plan for my children's future? I find energy to catch one more plane, give one more speech, make one more call when I remember that I am one small part of God's great adventure, and therefore it all has meaning. And

I am grateful that God has powerful arms to lift us. Because if I have learned nothing else along the route we travel, it is this: Pilgrims stumble.

Realizing that we stumble from time to time I've come with this request: I would like you to apply strong moral leadership to your institution's response to AIDS.

The religious community in this nation has, at best, a spotty record with regard to living out their own faiths when confronting AIDS. The Jewish community in which I was raised has for centuries championed the protection of those most vulnerable in society; with the smoke of the ovens still floating over us, it is hard to imagine how we could be so slow to respond to this epidemic. The Christian community was born into a manger of oppression and was nurtured on a gospel of compassion; how, then, could the doors to great cathedrals swing shut when those who were dying begged for grace? There are congregations of many faiths which have kept alive their ancient confessions and cared for those with AIDS. But we know them by name, because they have been so few. And their messages of hope and grace have been drowned out by the slogans of heretics who dress their evil political rhetoric in the language of faith and make God the author of this plague. If AIDS were indeed the judgment of God, it would not infect the pilgrim band; it would, instead, rain down on those who jeer and curse the pilgrims. And it would rain hardest on those who hurl their judgments from temples and pulpits.

The great faith represented here today has a tradition of holy spokespersons, prophets of God who took hard messages home to their own people. I want to encourage you to do that today. You know about stigma and discrimination, about those who live in fear and die alone. You know, too, about the profound absence of concern hundreds of thousands of deaths have evoked. I would like to hear your voice there, within the religious community you represent. I do not want you to leave your job to call for justice; I want you to do what you do best, justly. I do not want you to stop being a Catholic institution of healing; I want Catholic institutions to be known for grace.

Political, economic, social and scientific goals are all important in the struggle against AIDS. But so is spirituality. So is morality. So is a sharp and biting ethic. If you are in a position to elevate spirituality, press moral claims, establish ethical standards—the place we need you most, I am convinced, is where you are. Not on the streets or in the Congress, but in the board room and the classroom. Thoughtful politicians can call Americans to live responsibly in the neighborhoods and cities; but only a courageous prophet can call her people to live responsibly *in coram Deo*, in the face of God.

Of course we need credible legislation; pray and call for good legislation—but do it from the framework of your faith. Of course we need a cure and adequate care; work for scientific and economic support—but do it from the context of Catholic healthcare where the gospel is your tool. Let the core of your policies be the essence of your faith. Blow hard on ancient embers and let them burn brightly in the night of AIDS. We will never have enough support until the epidemic is conquered. But the barriers between the community of faith and the community of need must be taken down if we are to move forward.

In one sense, this is a simple call: Do what you do best. It's what I encourage people to do in every community I visit.

But here, today, it has special meaning. Because it takes special courage to speak prophetic words to the board of directors which wields financial and political power over us. It takes integrity on the border of heroism to challenge the priorities within our religious bureaucracies. Still, this is what I ask you to consider.

Jewish tradition contains many lessons regarding the prophets. One is: The prophets spoke for God. Another is: The prophets were often killed. I respect both lessons and trust you do as well. But pilgrims know that life presents difficult choices. If we have responded to a call from

God to make God's voice our own, then our integrity is found in our obedience. In this context, whether we obey is a matter for our choice; whether we are comfortable, that is God's choice.

Ignoring for a moment the Houston Astrodome and televised appearances, I've spoken to perhaps 100,000 people in person during the past year. Of those, I think I've probably hugged 10,000.

But standing out from all of them are the embraces with those who represent God. I could tell you today where they were, what they looked like, and what they said. Two little Sisters of Mercy who promised me prayers and then hugged me, both at the same time, one from each side, whispering in Latin a prayer I did not know. The pastor who'd introduced me to his congregation, but met me in the back of the sanctuary crying for a wife I did not know had died so recently. The African-American teacher who broke through a noisy swarm of high school students and began imploring God's grace in a teenaged bedlam.

What's unique about these hugs is that they were empowering. Here were arms like those of God, able to lift me when I was a stumbling pilgrim. Here were embraces filled with a strength unavailable to test tubes and researchers, a courage unattainable through psychological discipline or social convention, a hope that cannot be expressed apart from faith. Here is the difference between that healthcare conceived in a laboratory and that which is born in hope of a resurrection. This is the power that *you* possess, if you are indeed God's vessel filled with grace, and that *we* cannot live without.

For stumbling pilgrims kicking dust along the road to AIDS, to be empowered not only by hugs but also by heroic leadership is a great hope. Some of my fellow pilgrims no longer look eagerly toward the doors of temples when they trudge by; they look down when slouching past the church, expecting more trouble than grace. But you who are healers identified with the church, you could change that, if you wished. It does not require that you stand on the front porch as the pilgrim band moves past. Nor am I sure that by mounting a high pulpit, singing a loud song, or delivering a sermon you will catch the eye of many who've grown weary.

But this would do the trick: Push open the doors which have stood between God's uninfected people and his infected children. . .and come out. Come out as one who speaks for God. Don't wait any longer. Bring the healing gospel to the staggering pilgrimage. Pray with us. Laugh and weep with us. Heal us. Taste our hunger and thirst for a communion with God. Encourage the strong, embrace the weak, and cradle those who are dying. And, for me, look around the pilgrim band to see if you spot God—and point me in the right direction.

If, walking with the pilgrims, you find that on occasion your faith tires under the weight of the virus and your hope thins when watching others wither; if you discover that the pilgrimage toward AIDS is hard and, turning to ask about a rest, *you* stumble? It's all right. It's all right. It only means that now you, too, could pause along the way to AIDS and say, "We pilgrims. . . ."

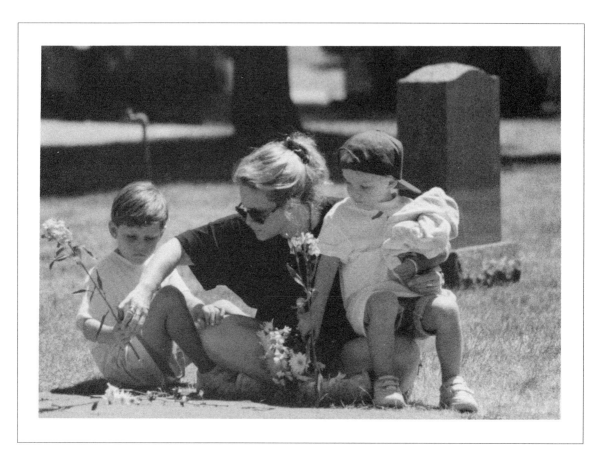

Waiting for Leadership

———————— o ————————

National Commission on AIDS
Washington, D.C.
June 28, 1993

More than a dozen years into the epidemic, the mandate of the National Commission on AIDS expired on a note of frustration and uncertainty. A news conference was called to mark the occasion—June 28, 1993—and Commissioners were asked to speak.

June had been a devastating month. After selling my home in Florida, the home I'd hoped for in the Washington area wasn't available, so I was moving everything twice—household and children, studio and offices—first to Michigan for the summer, and then to Washington. With life in chaos, Brian turned desperately ill and wanted to see me. I went to Boston.

First I was with Brian when he died. Then I was with the children at Brian's grave. Then I was in front of the micro-

203

phones in Washington where, emotionally shaken, I stumbled through this speech.

I did not give this speech out of some sense of civic duty, to finish my term as Commissioner with proper protocol. I spoke this time because I wanted to tell someone, anyone, everyone, that this is what the epidemic is like: It kills children's parents. It rips apart families. It hurts. It makes us all cry. I wanted people who measure diseases by statistics to know that Brian was no statistic, and neither are Max and Zack, and neither am I.

I will kneel with my sons in the fresh dirt of their father's grave, writing their names "for daddy," because I am their mother. But also because I am their mother, I am not willing to do it silently. So help me God, I am going to speak out. Occasionally with tears but mostly, I hope, with love.

My tenure on the Commission has been brief—it ends when the Commission adjourns, just before my eighth month in office. I want to use my last opportunity on this stage to make a few personal appeals.

To President and Mrs. Clinton, and those working with them to reform our nation's health policies, I promise every support, constant prayer and urgent vigilance. Though the Commission is adjourning, the commissioners live on in hope and concern. And we are, frankly, desperate for national leadership in the arena of AIDS. Where once there was hope perhaps too great or expectations perhaps too high, now there is suspicion—perhaps too deep. The air in the AIDS community is thick with the fear of broken promises.

On November 17, 1992, when I assumed my Commission chair, this is what I said to the previous Administration; I believe, respectfully, that it would also be my counsel to you. "We must speak thoughtfully, boldly, and consistently. . . . If we are silenced; if we shade the truth for political or personal gain; if we lower our voice when we hear the distant thunder of a political storm—then we have failed not only at public policy but, worse, at public trust."

And so my first appeal is to you, Mr. President: For the sake of millions of Americans dying and grieving—but more, for the sake of the nation itself—remember the promise of leadership, and lead.

To Christine Gebbie, named last week as "our nation's first AIDS Policy Coordinator," I offer publicly what I have promised her privately: My absolute support for every effort to find a cure, stop the spread, relieve the suffering, and care for the afflicted.

We on the Commission take our leave just as you take up the torch. I leave wishing you courage. When I came last fall, I said that "to press for better legislation without calling for greater dignity; to ask for more funds for HIV-positive citizens without challenging the immorality of the abuse they routinely suffer—to issue brave calls for government action without equally courageous calls to our fellow-citizens would call into question our own understanding of the issues." I believed it then. I still believe it now.

Therefore, I offer the same appeal to you, Christine, as to the President: Lead. Stand up and speak for those hundreds of thousands whose voices have been stilled. Speak gently of comfort to the grieving and quietly, with hope, for the dying. But speak boldly, loudly, to the nation. Be obsessed by your conscience; hate prejudice, love compassion, teach dignity, and do not fear losing when you go to battle for those with so little left to lose. In a word: Lead.

The gavel will sound, the cameras will go off, we'll shake hands all around and go home. But for some of us, going home is an odyssey into an uncertain future.

I spent last week at the bedside of the man with whom I shared two sons and eventually one virus. I've come from Brian's funeral. I spent last Saturday holding our sons at his graveside, writing our names in freshly turned dirt, drying their tears while struggling to see through my own, trying to make sense out of a five-year-old's grief and a three-year-old's questions.

The Commission is packing up and going home. And so am I. But I will not go passively, or quietly. When next my children stand at a parent's grave, they may be old enough to ask whether the nation cares. God help the person who needs to answer them. I am going to ask for leadership today, and again tomorrow, and I'm going to raise my voice each time I ask, until those who have asked for our confidence have earned it—by leading.

Let me be clear: It is not the AIDS community itself which is desperate for leadership, it's the nation at large. Those who imagine that this is someone else's problem, someone else's disease—these are people who need leaders, or they will surely die. The senator who compares HIV-positive immigrants with infected fruit; the preacher who regards the virus as God's good idea—these justify our call for leadership.

Most of all, the nation needs moral leadership. Without it, we will perish; with it, there is hope. Morally it is no more possible to think of this as a crisis for the infected than it is to think of slavery as an African-American problem, the holocaust as a Jewish problem, or abuse as a child's problem. When that message finds a leader to deliver it convincingly, we will begin to understand, as a nation, that this is our crisis. Perhaps then, for the first time, we will address it with the moral persuasion needed to wage, and win, a war.

I need to go home and answer hard questions from two children. But *someone* needs to lead.

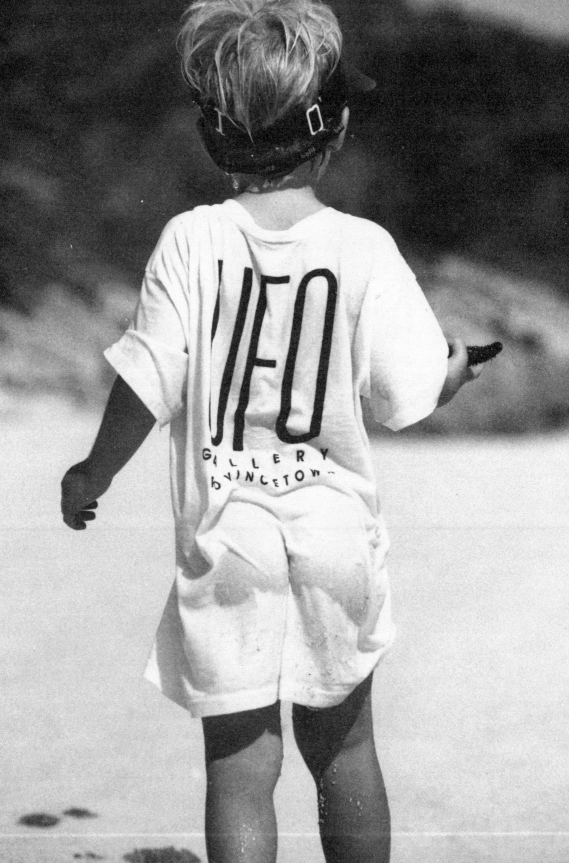

Notebook

———————o———————

It was a busy year, laying the groundwork for the Family AIDS Network by demonstrating its mission in communities across the country while simultaneously planning the organization's future.

From April, 1992, two months after I'd first told my story publicly, through June, 1993, when the National Commission on AIDS adjourned, we visited more than fifty communities. Variations of excerpts published in this book were sometimes included in addresses to other groups as well.

Palm Beach, Florida, Palm Beach Medical Society Auxiliary, Wednesday, April 1, 1992

New York City, AmFAR Award of Courage, Monday, April 13, 1992

Livonia, Michigan, Livonia Churchhill High School, Wednesday, April 15, 1992

Palm Beach County Community College, Wednesday, April 22, 1992

New York City, Mothers' Voices Luncheon, Monday, May 4, 1992

Boca Raton, Florida, Pine Crest School, Friday, May 8, 1992

Bloomfield Hills, Michigan, Julie Cummings's Coffee, Monday, May 11, 1992

Bloomfield Hills, Michigan, Cranbrook Schools, Monday, May 11, 1992

Salt Lake City, Testimony before the Republican Platform Committee, Tuesday, May 26, 1992

Boca Raton, Florida, AIDS Awareness Seminar for Parents, Monday, June 1, 1992

Detroit, WDIV/TV 4 Mary Fisher Documentary, Monday, June 8, 1992

Dearborn, Michigan, Michigan Women's Foundation Benefit Dinner, Tuesday, June 9, 1992

Columbus, Ohio, Columbus Cares Entertainment Benefit Red Ribbon Award, Saturday, June 13, 1992

Kansas City, Missouri, National Commission on AIDS, Monday, June 15, 1992

West Palm Beach, Florida, Heart Strings, Monday, June 22, 1992

Atlanta, Georgia, Heart Strings Final Performance, Friday, June 26, 1992

Various Cities, OpEd Column, Week of July 20, 1992

Amsterdam, VIII International Conference on AIDS/HIV STD World Congress, Thursday, July 23, 1992

Houston, The Republican National Convention, Wednesday, August 19, 1992

Detroit, AIDS Consortium of Southeastern Michigan, Tuesday, September 15, 1992

Santa Fe, New Mexico, Walk for Life, Saturday, October 3, 1992

Washington, D.C., The Names Project Memorial Quilt, Friday, October 9, 1992

Washington, D.C., 1992 National Skills Building Conference, Saturday, October 10, 1992

Charlotte, North Carolina, Myers Park Presbyterian Church, Sunday, October 11, 1992

Concord, North Carolina, National Day of Prayer for People Living with HIV/AIDS, All Saint's Episcopal Church, Sunday, October 11, 1992

Charlotte, North Carolina, Community Leadership Luncheon, Monday, October 12, 1992

Greensboro, North Carolina, Christ United Methodist Church, Monday, October 12, 1992

Greensboro, North Carolina, Community Leader Forum, Tuesday, October 13, 1992

Greensboro, North Carolina, Education Forum, Tuesday, October 13, 1992

Boston, Dana-Farber Cancer Institute Annual Meeting, Sunday, October 25, 1992

West Palm Beach, Florida, Walk for Life, Sunday, November 1, 1992

Palm Beach, Florida, Planned Parenthood, Thursday, November 5, 1992

Van Nuys, California, Church of the Valley, Sunday, November 8, 1992

Rancho Mirage, California, Betty Ford Center Workshops, Wednesday and Thursday, November 11-12, 1992

Rancho Mirage, California, Betty Ford Center Alumni Dinner, Saturday, November 14, 1992

Washington, D.C., National Commission on AIDS, Tuesday, November 17, 1992

Cedar City, Utah, Southern Utah University, Thursday, November 19, 1992

Salt Lake City, Eighth Annual Utah Women's Conference, Friday, November 20, 1992

New York City, *Town & Country* 1992 Most Generous American Award Dinner, Wednesday, December 2, 1992

New York City, The Nightingale-Bamford School Assemblies, Wednesday, December 2, 1992, and Wednesday, December 16, 1992

Memphis, The Women's Coalition of Memphis, Thursday, January 14, 1993

Memphis, Second Presbyterian Church, Sunday, January 17, 1993

Austin, Texas, LBJ High School, Tuesday, February 2, 1993

Austin, Texas, Junior League of Austin, Tuesday, February 2, 1993

Hartford, Connecticut, Connecticut Forum, Saturday, February 6, 1993

San Diego, University of San Diego, Monday, February 15, 1993

San Diego, The Women's Coalition of University of San Diego, Monday, February 15, 1993

Los Angeles, UCLA, Tuesday, February 16, 1993

Hamden, Connecticut, National Institute for Community Health Education, Wednesday, March 3, 1993

Troy, Michigan, Troy-Athens High School, Monday, March 8, 1993

Ann Arbor, Michigan, University of Michigan Social Work Conference, Tuesday, March 9, 1993

Ann Arbor, Michigan, Huron High School, Tuesday, March 9, 1993

Austin, Texas, Hyde Park Baptist Church, Wednesday, March 10, 1993

Boston, New England Hospital and Health Care Foundation 1993 Annual Convention, Thursday, April 1, 1993

Salem, Massachusetts, Salem State College, Thursday, April 1, 1993

Cleveland, Ohio, Alliance to the American Dental Association 1993 Annual Leadership Conference, Thursday, April 1, 1993

Detroit, National Op-Ed Page Editors Conference, Sunday, April 18, 1993

Big Rapids, Michigan, Ferris State University, Tuesday, April 20, 1993

Grand Rapids, Michigan, Grand Rapids Press Bob Day Annual Dinner, Wednesday, April 21, 1993

Grand Rapids, Michigan, Forest Hills High Schools, Thursday, April 22, 1993

Grand Rapids, Michigan, Planned Parenthood, Thursday, April 22, 1993

Grand Rapids, Michigan, Grand Rapids AIDS Foundation Reception, Thursday, April 22, 1993

Grand Rapids, Michigan, Ecumenical AIDS Service, St. James Catholic Church, Thursday, April 22, 1993

Detroit, Hospice of Southeastern Michigan Crystal Rose Award Dinner, Saturday, April 24, 1993

New York City, Cornell University Medical Center Grand Rounds, Thursday, April 29, 1993

New York City, Seamen's Church Institute, Tuesday, May 6, 1993

Detroit, Shape Up Michigan Rally, Friday, May 14, 1993

Detroit, University of Detroit Mercy, Saturday, May 15, 1993

New York City, Americans for Medical Progress Educational Foundation Dinner, Tuesday, May 18, 1993

New Britain, Connecticut, Rock for Hope Softball Game, Saturday, May 23, 1993

Hartford, Connecticut, Trinity College Commencement, Sunday, May 23, 1993

Fairfield, Connecticut, The Stewart B. McKinney Foundation Fifth Annual Awards Dinner, Tuesday, June 1, 1993

New York City, World War Against AIDS Rally, Bryant Park, Sunday, June 6, 1993

Mamaroneck, New York, Mamaroneck High School, Monday, June 7, 1993

New Orleans, 78th Annual Catholic Health Association Membership Assembly, Tuesday, June 8, 1993

Washington, D.C., National Commission on AIDS, Monday, June 28, 1993

A few written pieces from my notebook of the past year do not qualify as speeches but may, for one reason or another, interest readers.

In workshops and speeches and informal remarks, when I've believed my audience could use some basic information about the AIDS epidemic, I've frequently made some or all of a dozen points.

To be helpful in the fight with HIV/AIDS, we need to know the basic facts. If I were to quickly scan just a dozen facts, they would be these:

1. HIV—the human immunodeficiency virus—breaks down the human immune system in ways we do not fully understand. There is no vaccine to prevent it, and currently no cure once you contract it.

2. AIDS—acquired immunodeficiency syndrome—is not a different disease than HIV. It is just the name we give to the condition which results when HIV has worn down the immune system to the point where other diseases can attack. AIDS is really "late stage HIV."

3. People do not die of AIDS. They grow progressively weaker owing to HIV until they enter that stage of infection called AIDS, and then other infectious diseases kill them. It could be cancer or brain infection; most often it's pneumonia or, sometimes, tuberculosis.

4. In national statistics, people with HIV alone are not ordinarily included in AIDS numbers. Good scientific and political reasons account for this, but it leaves a dangerous sense of false safety for the casual listener, because for every AIDS case that is reported, up to ten HIV infections exist.

5. More than 200,000 Americans have died of AIDS-related causes. It took ten years for the first 100,000 to die; it took less than two

years for the second 100,000. Because this is an epidemic, not a flat-rate disease, it is charted with an upward spiral.

6. To date, everyone with HIV appears to develop AIDS. That's what makes the HIV statistics important. As of today, the probabilities of developing AIDS if you are HIV-positive are about 100%.

7. We do not have a precise count on HIV-positive Americans, but credible estimates suggest there are one-and-a-half or two million people now infected with the virus in the U.S.

8. Because HIV can exist without symptoms for as much as a decade, unless we are aware that somewhere in our lives we were at risk, we may be HIV-positive. If we remain ignorant of this, and of how to protect others, we may infect others.

9. Most people who die of complications resulting from AIDS are in the prime of their life at a time when, ordinarily, they would not have required extensive health care. Unless there is a cure, AIDS patients will add significantly to the stress on America's already overloaded health care systems before the year 2000.

10. This is not a disease limited to gay men or needle-using drug addicts. It is historical coincidence that the disease spread first in gay communities in America. But the virus has jumped all fences now. Worldwide, it is overwhelmingly a heterosexually transmitted disease. In the U.S., the fastest growing rates of infection are among women, children and adolescents.

11. Ten years ago, fewer than one in 100 Americans knew someone who was HIV positive. Five years ago, it was one in 20. Today, it is one in four. In 36 months, it'll be a perfect one-to-one ratio.

12. I do not fit all "standard" categories, but I am HIV-positive.

*When the Michigan Women's Foundation asked if I would
introduce June Osborn, M.D.—then Professor and Dean of
the School of Public Health at the University of Michigan,
and Chair of the National Commission on AIDS—to receive
an award in 1992, I was delighted to accept. This is a woman
the world should know.*

When Yale University bestowed an honorary doctorate of
medical sciences on Dr. June Osborn on May 25, 1992, they
offered her an elegant tribute for "reminding us passionately and
poetically of how much we have lost personally and as a society,"
inspiring us "in these tragic times" with compassion.

Yale was right in what it said of this woman. As our world
braces for perhaps 100 million new HIV infections in the coming
decade, it looks to her for hope and for direction. And the world
is right in looking to this woman; there will be no leader with
finer insight, greater courage, or deeper compassion.

The notable Dr. Osborn praised by Yale and admired by the
world is also the June Osborn who did not enter my life on a
public stage; she came to me quietly, embracing me, encouraging me to find my own insight, develop my own courage, and find
my own voice of compassion. Both in the quiet hours of privacy
and in the glare of public moments, I've been comforted by this
marvelous healer.

Watching her with presidents and prime ministers, who
would suspect either the humor or the shyness of this woman?
I felt both recently when she and I were meeting with parents
of some high schoolers. After answering the umpteenth question about attitudes toward sexuality, she leaned over and
quietly asked, "Should I tell them that I travel the world

discussing sexual intercourse but am embarrassed by MTV?"

Listening to her address massive conventions and academic conferences, could anyone imagine her at home with her garden? See her delicate needlepointing done with a doctor's hands and an artist's soul? Hear her wise counsel to children she loves intensely enough to shield them from the glare of her own public limelight? In these things we share—from needlepointing to affection for our children—we have been women together, mothers together, friends.

At a glance, June Osborn could pass for Golda Meir come-back-to-life. Some people in high offices, who've experienced her tough-mindedness in response to their soft-mindedness, might think there are other resemblances between those two women. I suspect that after God made June Osborn, She (God) said to the angels, "One of these will be enough to change the world."

History has been changed by her tenacity, while many of us have been touched by her tenderness. Because, like me, she is a woman gripped by AIDS—gripped differently, perhaps, but clearly my dear fellow-traveler on this sometimes difficult road. This is a woman, after all, who so savors life and so respects it, that she cannot endure the loss of even one. And so she campaigns tirelessly to save millions of lives, while she hugs us one at a time.

The world is right, June, in honoring you. Yale and the Michigan Women's Foundation are right in paying you tribute. It's true that both your passion and your poetry have made our times less tragic. I know that intimately, because you have helped me make of my life not a tragedy but a testimony.

To honor you is noble. To introduce you is delightful. But to love you, June, and to be loved by you, is by far the greatest joy.

Organizers of the 1992 Amsterdam "World Congress" requested an op-ed column to be run in selected papers the week before the conference opened in The Netherlands. Mine ran in a number of newspapers under the heading, "Finding An Expert's Voice."

Five months after telling the world that I am HIV-positive, I'll visit Amsterdam to address the VIII International Conference on AIDS/HIV STD World Congress. I'll speak as "an expert," according to advance publicity, one of several such experts participating in a Roundtable on "the experience of persons living with HIV/AIDS."

This is still all new to me. Television studios and the White House are professionally comfortable territory; I've spent years at work in both. For near-perfect professional contentment, put me in the quiet of my home studio for a day and let me do my art. But surround me with world-class doctors and scientists, epidemiologists and researchers, heavily-degreed people who speak a language of biotechnology we lay people can barely grasp—such a setting is not calculated to make me feel like an expert.

The "expertise" planners believe I can bring, of course, is not drawn from research or science or abstract study. They've asked me to speak as one who lives with HIV, one who knows the virus more intimately than scientifically. They want me to answer the question, What is it like to live as an infected person?

I've not yet decided what I'll say. Perhaps I should tell them the virus is just a part of the human existence. Some people wrestle with emotional illness, others with wayward children or addictions or cancer or lonesomeness. As it has happened, I wrestle with HIV. They have their burdens. I have mine.

Or, if it would help anyone, I could talk about the calm I experience because of my conviction that Divine purpose infuses all that happens, including what happens to and through me. If it would not seem self-centered or foolish, I'd tell them that though I detest this virus and what it will do to me, I believe the virus has been used to call me to my place in world history.

Maybe I should talk about pain. I could tell them of my relief when first I knew that neither of my children were infected, and how ecstacy gave way to agony when first I calculated the odds on living to see my two-year-old, Zachary, as a teenager.

Would it help if I showed the hurt I felt when otherwise-thoughtful, decent and educated adults doubted my four-year-old (Max) should hug a teddy bear for fear that, because he lives with me, they'd be put at risk?

Or does speaking of pain merely make me sound like a hapless victim?

Perhaps I should prepare to speak uniquely as an American. After all, this is a World Congress and I attend wearing the badge of my nation. To experience HIV as an American mom is quite different than to experience it as, say, a Ugandan child or an Asian prostitute.

Experts in the arithmetic of plagues warn us to brace for over 100,000,000 HIV infections around the year 2000. America is drenched with wealth and knowledge, and America has long told the world that our values are the ones which should be imitated. The unfortunate truth is, however, that our nation has been slow to rally its wealth or its knowledge to this crisis. Staring at a hundred million faces which belong to my fellow-travelers, no matter their race or gender or color or nationality, what should I say of American priorities?

I am off to Amsterdam to say something of living with HIV. If I told nothing but the stark truth, it would go something like this: I hate HIV because disease and death are brutal enemies. I love my children, family and friends. I intend to live with courage and with integrity. And I cannot explain why American priorities seem so little affected by millions of us, here and abroad, whose lives are being smothered by HIV/AIDS.

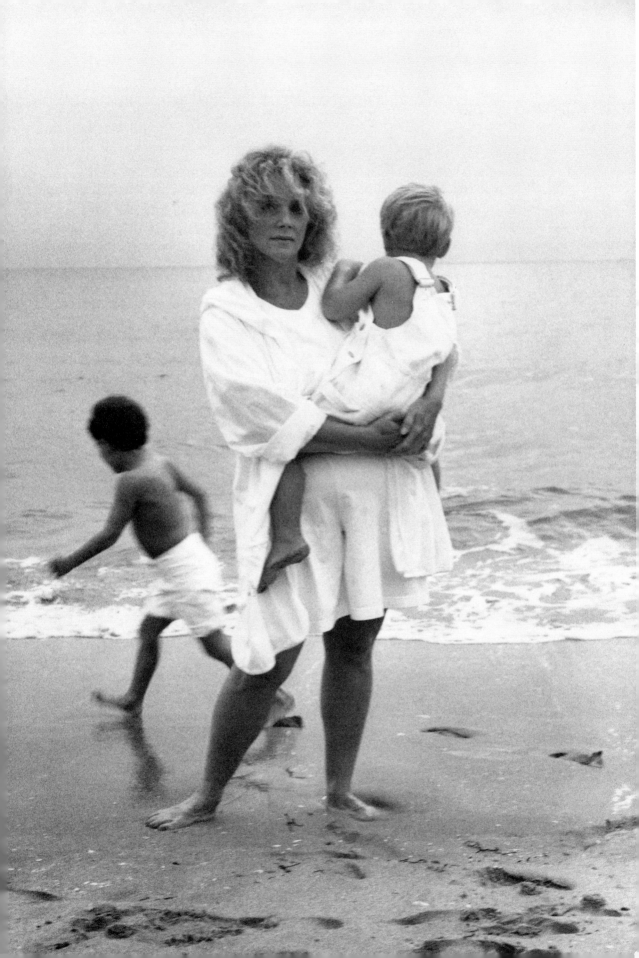